Stop Stuffing Your Face

How You Can Control Emotional Eating and Overcome Food Addiction

Jason Newman

© Copyright 2022 - All rights reserved.

The content contained within this book may not be reproduced, duplicated or transmitted without direct written permission from the author or the publisher.

Under no circumstances will any blame or legal responsibility be held against the publisher, or author, for any damages, reparation, or monetary loss due to the information contained within this book, either directly or indirectly.

Legal Notice:

This book is copyright protected. It is only for personal use. You cannot amend, distribute, sell, use, quote or paraphrase any part, or the content within this book, without the consent of the author or publisher.

Disclaimer Notice:

Please note the information contained within this document is for educational and entertainment purposes only. All effort has been executed to present accurate, up to date, reliable, complete information. No warranties of any kind are declared or implied.

Readers acknowledge that the author is not engaged in the rendering of legal, financial, medical or professional advice. The content within this book has been derived from various sources. Please consult a licensed professional before attempting any techniques outlined in this book.

By reading this document, the reader agrees that under no circumstances is the author responsible for any losses, direct or indirect, that are incurred as a result of the use of the information contained within this document, including, but not limited to, errors, omissions, or inaccuracies.

Table of Contents

Introduction

Chapter 1: What is Emotional Eating?

    How Do You Know if You're an Emotional Eater?

        The Emotional Eating Cycle

        The Effects on Your Body

Chapter 2: Reasons That Lead to Emotional Eating

    Stress

        Past Traumas

        Depression and Low Self-Esteem

        Boredom and Reward

    Is Emotional Eating Bad?

Chapter 3: Physical Hunger vs. Emotional Hunger

    How Our Ancestors Treated Food and Eating

        The Seven Types of Hunger

Chapter 4: How Do Hormones Play a Role?

    Ghrelin

    Leptin

    Insulin

    Peptide YY

    Cortisol

    Estrogen and Progesterone

    Ways to Fix the Hormones that Control Your Weight

Chapter 5: Importance of Diet and Exercise

    The Importance of Nutrients

    Staying Hydrated

    Making It a Lifestyle Change

Chapter 6: The Effects of Advertising

    Fast-Food Chains

    Advertisement and Body Image

Chapter 7: Controlling Emotional Eating

- Mindful Eating
  - Change Your Habits, Change Your Mind
  - Self-Care
  - Emotional Health
- Conclusion
- Afterword
- References

Introduction

The monthly budget meeting has crept up again; the one where your boss is nice enough to supply coffee, donuts, muffins—typically a tray full of carbs. Psychologists say anything that's free or feels like a good deal, especially when it's in a work environment, and if you're feeling underappreciated in any way, can feel like an extra perk. Stress and boredom are two of the top reasons people emotionally eat, and those are both felt most often at work. Factor in the social aspect of eating with co-workers, and you have a lot of influence on your eating habits at work.

You're at a birthday party, and the snack table is calling your name. You know you want to change some of your habits and break free from the hold food has on you, and maybe you just want to start eating healthy. It's impossible not to say no when everyone in the room is partaking. Okay, maybe just one donut, one piece of cake... That turns into a full plate of junk food, and you leave feeling full but still empty inside. Next week you have to struggle with it all over again on that 30th wedding anniversary...

Do those scenarios sound all too familiar to you? Emotions can take over our reasoning when it comes to what we eat and how much. Emotions are something we can't necessarily control because they are the mind's automatic response to things in their environment. Sometimes impulses run high, and they can be hard to reign in. That doesn't mean you can't work at trying to control your emotions or conquer them in a healthier way that doesn't involve obsessing over food or thinking food is the only outlet.

Turning to food whenever you have an emotional high or low can affect your health in many negative ways. If we eat too frequently, even without being physically hungry, or consume too many calories, that can lead to weight gain and, eventually, it could lead to obesity. Obesity is on the rise, and people who struggle with their relationship with food might develop it over a long period. Over 300,000 deaths in the US a year are attributed to obesity (Lehnardt. 2017). It's a harsh reality that comes with a poor diet, processed foods, and an unhealthy lifestyle. According to the World Health Organization, there are around two billion adults overweight, of whom 650 million are considered to be affected by obesity (World Obesity Federation, 2016). As one of the most important public health crises, obesity is a growing concern, not to be ignored.

The way food is portrayed has been shaped in people's thinking patterns and habits since biblical times with Adam and Eve and the abundance of food in the Garden of Eden. The idea of Heaven as a place where food was plentiful and the promise of a land of milk and honey seems all too descriptive of "food heaven." The Bible is also filled with food imagery and almost every biblical event of any importance was accompanied with a meal, food also often being a sacrificial offering to God.

There are so many ways to get sucked in these days with advertisements for food and restaurants shown every time you turn on a screen. It's tough to avoid the temptations constantly surrounding your daily tasks and activities. Driving on the highway, every other road billboard is for a fast-food restaurant, enticing you to hit their drive-thru. There is a fast-food restaurant on every block, and even though you know you'll regret it afterward, how can you resist a satisfying combo meal? You can't even go into the gas station to pay for your fill-up without being bombarded by the candy and snacks surrounding the front area where you need to pay. It's even harder to go to the grocery store for your weekly list of groceries. If you have made a list beforehand of what you plan to cook for the week, it is hard not to be sidetracked by the ice cream aisle and the countless ways they sneak in a display of the newest flavor of chip. These distractions make it hard not to bring home the kinds of snacks and sweets you might turn to for comfort.

Emotional eating has played a large role in the way you think about food. Have you ever sat down and eaten an entire bag of chips and weren't even hungry? How do you even know if you're emotionally eating? It's not just about feeling sad and indulging in a tub of ice cream. Sometimes we celebrate by going out for an indulgent dinner, or maybe we have gotten stressed out from day to day and feel better after our favorite sweet. If you are eating to feel better, then you are emotionally eating. That can lead to overeating, which will lead to weight gain and the other health concerns that go along with extra weight gain.

If you can identify the ways in which you are finding food that makes you feel better in your life, then you can stop the cycle of emotional eating. It's about learning to accept your feelings and own them, even if they are tougher emotions. There are many other things you can be doing in your life to stop emotional eating, and they are laid out in this book.

My passion is helping others with their struggles. I hope this book can find you some relief in the fact that you are not alone with your struggles, and you can get through them. Some of my other written works include *How to Control Your Alcohol Consumption; Learn to Drink Responsibly So That You Can Enjoy a Drink Rather Than Depend on It*.

Chapter 1: What is Emotional Eating?

You don't always eat to satisfy your physical feelings of hunger and receive nutrition for your bodies. With emotional eating, you are filling an emotional need instead of the needs of your body. It may not even be necessarily a negative emotion. There are positive emotions you may feel that you relate to eating. Most foods you might find comforting, or you enjoy while experiencing different emotions, are the unhealthiest, and you turn to them when you feel different emotions, not necessarily sadness but even as a reward or sheer boredom. Finding comfort in foods you enjoy is common. Research shows that about 75% of all of our eating is emotionally driven, but it is best to deal with your emotions more healthily and productively (Emotional Eating: What It Is and Tips to Manage It, 2021). Turning to food for comfort is not a long-term solution and will only make you feel worse afterwards. You will feel guilty if you overindulge, and after time, the consequences will show in your waistline, and you will most likely still have those negative feelings.

Emotional eating is not always caused by one single thing, but several situations in your life could affect how much food you eat, how often, and whether it is nutritious for your body. Emotional eating is not necessarily the desire to eat but the emotions you feel that lead you to want to eat, even if you aren't hungry. Negative emotions may lead to a feeling of emptiness or an emotional void. That is why people feel that food is a way to fill that void and create a false feeling of 'fullness' or temporary wholeness. You may feel physically full, but something is still missing in your life, and you continue to use food to fill it. The foods that emotional eaters crave are often referred to as comfort foods, like chocolate, sweets, ice cream, pizza, fast food, or salty snacks such as chips.

Emotional eating is not necessarily the same as binge eating, but they can correlate and end up on a continuum. Binge eating is a more extreme version of emotional eating, but emotional eating can lead to binge eating. Binge eaters often feel like they are out of control and continue to eat, even until they feel nauseous. Some who emotionally eat are able to get over it and not continue to do it, but when you can't control your eating based on your emotions, you may have to take a look at yourself and the relationship you have with food.

How Do You Know if You're an Emotional Eater?

We may all have gone through emotional eating at some point in our lives. Nearly 2.5 million adults in the United States today suffer from compulsive overeating, with probably many more unreported cases (Celes, n.d.). Some people might use it as a coping mechanism for one or multiple dealings in their lives or the emotions they can't control. Do you eat to satisfy your hunger? Do you eat when you are feeling sad, in pain, majorly stressed out, or bored? Do you feel better when you have eaten to the point of being stuffed? Do you feel like you are in control more when you can have your favorite snack? Do you reward yourself with a piece of chocolate, or do you eat the whole bar? Can you have a handful of chips to satisfy your snack attack, or do you need to demolish the entire bag? These are all important questions if you think you eat emotionally. You may not even realize you are doing it, but it's important to be aware of it, aware of how often these actions occur, and that when a craving doesn't come from hunger, you can never satisfy it.

Here are some signs that you are an emotional eater:

- **You eat when you are feeling stressed:** Whether you are bombarded with tasks at work or your kids are stressing you out, they all make you want to eat.
- **You eat in response to your emotions:** Whether you are feeling sad, annoyed, disappointed, angry, lonely, empty, anxious, tired, or bored, they are all emotional reasons for you to grab something to eat instead of being physically hungry.

- **You see comfort in your food:** You are not even sure why, but you are comforted by food and feeling full.
- **You can't lose weight because of your eating habits:** Most of the food you find comforting is high-calorie and unhealthy, so if you do try to work out, it seems to go unnoticed when you are consuming so many empty calories.
- **You eat to feel better or eat when you are happy:** It is not the same as having an appreciation for food, but you feel like you rely on it to feel happy, and you treat food as a positive companion, just like you would eat to celebrate something.
- **You eat when you aren't hungry:** You continue to think of food or consume it. Even though you are full, you can't seem to stop

yourself. Additionally, you can't wait until the next time you can eat, and you are constantly craving, counting down until the next meal.

The Emotional Eating Cycle

When you constantly use food as a coping mechanism, you might feel better, but the feeling won't last, and you will end up feeling worse than you did before you stuffed your face. It leads to an unwanted cycle.

1. Something internal or external happens in your environment that upsets you.
2. You are overwhelmed with the need to eat something unhealthy.
3. You eat until you are over-full.
4. You feel guilty for overeating and feel like you have no power over food.

5. Then it starts all over again, and the cycle continues.

When you use food to help conquer your emotions, the cycle repeats, and your health will continue to be affected. Eating empty calories and consuming more than you require equals added weight and other health issues.

Get into a new cycle of not giving in, and you will find yourself less dependent on food, less depressed, and realizing the power the emotional eating cycle has over you.

The Effects on Your Body

Those comfort foods that you often turn to when emotionally eating, usually convenience food, are typically high in chemical additives, hormones, sugar, salt, unhealthy fat, and calories, all of which can adversely affect your brain and overall health (Robinson et al., 2019). Consuming too many processed foods involves having an abundant amount of fat, sugar, and salt. The effects of that on your body can be extremely detrimental to your overall health. There are many other adverse effects of having too much fat, sugar, and salt in your diet:

1. **The effect on your cognitive abilities:** Only after a week, your brain is affected by a diet too high in fat, sugar, and salt.
2. **You constantly crave them more:** This becomes a vicious cycle of poor eating habits because your brain constantly craves fat, sugar, and salt, easily depending on these three things, becoming an addiction.
3. **It slows you down:** When you don't get enough vital nutrients from the food you eat, you start to feel sluggish and lethargic. Your

energy levels are going to be low if you consume high amounts of sugar. Cutting back is not going to be easy, so it's best to start out slowly.

4. **It can make you sick:** Your body shouldn't be depending on too much sugar and salt. When you aren't consuming enough healthy fats and nutrients, your immune system suffers, and that is the quickest way to get sick, even if it is just the common cold.

Scientists have found a certain part of the brain that affects sugar addiction and compulsive eating. This area of the brain is the pleasure center, and it is what contributes to addiction. It could be food, drugs, or anything that sends a message to your brain that you enjoyed it so much, you can't wait to have it again. Food has always been thought of as positive reinforcement, whether you are enjoying it or you even see an image of it. Because this is a chemical dependency, the incessant craving for unhealthy junk foods can be hard to ignore, and the power of the mind takes over the actions sometimes. Our brain associates these foods you really enjoy and continues to crave them. The best thing you can do is slowly wean off the amount of sugar you are consuming and find other healthier alternatives that you can still enjoy without feeling guilty or having too many processed foods.

It is a good idea to know the facts about overconsumption of fats, sugar, and salt. There was such a thing as the Einstein test. Back when Albert Einstein would invite potential colleagues or research assistants to dinner, he would watch intently on whether or not they seasoned their food before they even took a bite to figure out if it needed salt or pepper. He would dismiss them at once if they chose to season without tasting, assuming they lacked an open mind. This goes to show what someone could think of you and your seasoning habits, but more importantly, you don't always need to add salt to your food, so make sure you taste it, and chances are if you are out to eat, you don't need to add anymore.

Knowing the facts might help you understand, and you will be less likely to want to put so much of these harmful substances in your body. Of course, salt and sugar are both used in cooking and baking, so they are not volatile, but in high quantities over long periods of time, they can be. What do fat, salt, and sugar really do to your body?

Too much sodium, one of the components of salt, may cause hypertension, or high blood pressure. High blood pressure can cause a number of health complications, including heart disease and stroke. It can also cause water retention, which leads to excess bloating, increased swelling especially in the hands and feet, and can cause you to weigh more than usual. Certain cancers are linked to high salt consumption, like stomach cancer, by causing ulcers or inflammation of the stomach lining.

There are a lot more negative effects of too much sugar than you think. Too much sugar causes tooth decay and excess weight gain, which can lead to obesity. When you eat excess sugar, the extra insulin in your bloodstream can affect your arteries all over your body, and over time this can damage your heart. The effects it has on your brain and your mood is also not healthy. Sugar causes too much dopamine in your brain, that 'happy' hormone, and your brain senses that pleasure and constantly craves it again, becoming highly addictive just as any drug would. Too much sugar has been known to cause depression in some. That sugar crash you feel is often caused by having sugar earlier in the day, and if you continue to experience that crash, it affects your mood long-term. Too much sugar can cause inflammation, and that can affect your joints. It can also speed up the aging process on your skin. Fructose is processed in the liver, so too much sugar can be harmful to your liver. Not to mention your pancreas, which works when you eat food. With too much sugar, your pancreas has to pump out more insulin to balance the levels, and eventually, your overworked pancreas could cause type 2 diabetes. If left untreated, diabetes can severely damage your kidneys. It all circles back to the culprit, which is sugar.

When you emotionally eat, you are usually eating to the point you are stuffed, making you feel better. The foods that make you feel happy are the ones that taste the best and are usually the junk food type: high in fat and calories. Controlling your portions is important for proper digestion and, of course, keeping your weight in control. Consuming all these extra calories is bound to lead to weight gain, which, in turn, could also lead to obesity. Excessive weight gain and obesity can lead to many other health concerns we should be aware of, such as

1. **Increased risk of disease:** Heart disease, stroke, certain cancers, and type 2 diabetes are some of the risks of weight gain.

2. **Excess body fat:** If you don't balance out your calorie consumption with what you burn, you can gain weight and excess body fat. When you consume too many calories, your body will store it as fat. When you overeat, you are likely consuming more calories than you require.

3. **Nausea and indigestion:** Your stomach can only hold so much, and when you eat at a faster

pace, your stomach will reach capacity and could even make you vomit.

4. **Gas and bloating:** Large amounts of food entering your stomach at a fast rate can cause gas and bloating. Eating slower and waiting until after you eat to drink liquids does help.

5. **Brain function:** Studies have shown that over time, overeating can negatively affect the brain and cause a mental decline in older individuals.

6. **Tired and sluggish:** After eating a huge meal, your blood sugar drops, so after overeating, you are most likely to feel sleepy.

Reducing portion sizes, choosing more whole foods, and even talking to a dietician is best to avoid further complications with your overall health. This may be more of a challenge with all the reasons we have to emotionally eat circling our lives.

Chapter 2: Reasons That Lead to Emotional Eating

The contributing reason for emotional eating is just that—our emotions. What about some factors we may not think about or think are causing emotional eating?

Do you have a family member who shows you love by making your food? Do you do the same to others? Sometimes it's a nice gesture to make the host of a party a batch of cookies or bake a pie for someone we love, but it becomes more of an issue if that is the only way you feel you can express your love or affection for someone. If you have someone that constantly showers you with home-cooked, high-fat foods, they are acting as an enabler to you, and you might want to explain to them how you feel.

Exhaustion is a leading cause of emotional eating. You may not even realize you are contributing your emotional eating to being tired. Your pleasure center is more easily activated when you are sleep-deprived, so that is most likely why you want a greasy pizza or pack of donuts to pull through an all-nighter for work or school.

Even bonding with someone can drive you to emotional eating. Studies show people consume more food in front of a crowd, regardless of whether they are hungry at all (Higgs & Thomas, 2016). You might feel shy and awkward, so you see the food table and head there to keep your hands looking busy. You can walk around with a plate full of food and eventually will eat it all, hoping to strike up a conversation with someone.

Emotional eating could have started as young as a newborn baby. Nursing and feeding are correlated with love, comfort, and closeness. As a young child, when your parents used food to reward you, you learned to enjoy food as a means of pleasure and accomplishments. Rewarding you with food has always been the norm as small children and as you grew into your teens. It has never been looked at as a bad way of parenting, and the association with food and reward has not been a stranger to society. Your parents might have taken you for dinner when you had a good report card or celebrated the winning goal at your soccer game with ice cream. You will most likely take these traditions into adulthood, and the feeling of nostalgia will bring back these memories and habits.

Emotional eating can affect individuals of all ages. Many individuals don't admit their problem, so it is hard to know exactly how many people are affected by emotional eating. It may be researched that women are more affected by it, but that is only because many men don't want to admit they have a problem with food. There is nothing to be ashamed of, and there are all kinds of reasons that may be affecting the way you feel and think about food.

Men can be affected by emotional eating just as much if not more than women, but the stigma and stereotyping that encompasses weight gain and obesity are extremely biased. It is pretty evident that society has its own skewed opinions on weight for men and weight for women. In the entertainment business, movies and television shows applauded overweight men more than they do women. Women seem to be judged, ridiculed and shamed more than men do. It is more accepted for men to be overweight, and the woman is viewed as more unattractive. The common reasons you hear are something like, "men like their beer and watching their sports." It almost seems like men are given a free pass, excuses are made for them, and the judgment is not there or as harsh as it can be for women. Does this encourage men to eat whatever they want and gain weight as they please when women are considered lazy and unmotivated? Sadly, it seems to be more acceptable for men to be overweight than for women.

The way Hollywood movies have portrayed fat people, especially women, has normalized fat-shaming and made fat people the brunt of the jokes. There are many male celebrities out there who are overweight, but they are thought of as funny, cute, tough, and even handsome. In Hollywood, fat men can be powerful and sexy. There never seem to be roles like that for the opposite sex. There are celebrities that are known for their fat roles and have been told not to lose weight or they will never work in Hollywood again. The majority of the TV shows we see, adult cartoons, and movies have overweight men with unrealistically attractive wives, and no one seems to talk about how crazy that is and how that would never happen if the roles were reversed. When a female celebrity gains weight, even a small amount, everyone seems to notice, but the same is not true for Hollywood male celebrities.

What message is this sending? Not very positive ones at all. It makes it seem more acceptable for men to be overweight, so they don't have all the pressure to lose it. That makes it harder for men to take their weight seriously. According to research, the number of overweight men is growing much more than women. Between 1999 and 2000, there were more obese women than men. By the late 2000s, men had caught up to women and had started to inch past them in terms of overweight and obesity rates (Cathe, 2014). The focus needs to be put back on staying healthy and being conscious of a healthier lifestyle.

As a society, we have decidedly and correctly been accepting of gender preferences, sexual orientation, or marital status but still can't seem to accept people that are overweight and show compassion or kindness. Society and the public may think that your weight is something you choose to control with the amount of food you eat and the amount of exercise you get, but there are some individuals who are predisposed to obesity due to genetics. Globally, obesity has reached epidemic proportions with approximately 1.5 billion adults reaching the overweight or obese categories (Vitagene, 2018). Many of the skeptical people out there may believe that a person is overweight because they choose not to work out or eat too many calories and choose unhealthy foods. However, there are many people who have a genetic predisposition to be overweight, and it will be a constant struggle.

The idea of nature vs. nurture comes into play, and it is a fairly ongoing debate, but it is important to consider when it comes to obesity. Nature refers to all of the hereditary factors such as physical appearance and personality characteristics. Nurture focuses on more of the environmental aspects such as how you grew up, how you were raised, and other relationships along with social and cultural factors. The big debate is which factors have the most influence on your behaviors.

An individual's environment was believed to be more of a factor in weight gain and obesity, but now with DNA testing, genetics has become more of a consideration. It is important to understand the role genetics could play in the obesity epidemic. After much research, studies have come to show that body weight and obesity are 65-80% predetermined by a person's genetic makeup (Vitagene, 2018).

When it comes to genetics, researchers have focused on two types of obesity. Monogenic and polygenic. This is important to note because monogenic obesity refers to individuals who have certain mutations that cause obesity, and polygenic obesity refers to individuals who have combined effects of genetic variants. Polygenic obesity is more common among those with obesity. This means there could be several genes that contribute to leading causes of obesity, but that doesn't mean that individuals can't fight against the genetic predisposition to becoming obese.

With DNA testing, there are decisions you can make and steps you can take to find out what you can do to make better choices with nutrition, diet, and exercise. Just because you might have genetics telling you that you could become obese doesn't mean you have to let that happen. Only you can make the changes in your life to work with your body and be where you want to be with your weight and health. All of the important changes you make in your life are about being accountable and staying consistent. It's all about your lifestyle.

The link between income and obesity has also been thought to have an impact on the foods we choose and certain lifestyle choices. The cost to be healthy is much higher, and that includes food, gym passes, and other factors that add up to living a healthy lifestyle. There was a time when fast-food restaurants realized they should start making more healthy alternatives to their menu. The problem is the hype didn't compare to reality. The cost for a healthy salad was much higher than your average "value meal." There are places you can go and have a healthy green smoothie or a cold-pressed juice, but you are breaking the bank for the healthy alternative. The healthy alternative didn't last long, and the dollar menus live on strong.

The same goes for the grocery stores. Produce is on the rise, and the less expensive food that lives on the inside shelves is where a lot of people on a tight budget will turn. Eating healthier does not necessarily have to break the bank though. Certain healthy items you find at the supermarket can be more expensive, such as organic or gluten-free items, but that doesn't mean regular produce, lean meats, nuts, or healthy canned or frozen items can't be in your budget. This means obviously trying to stay away from overly processed foods full of preservatives and other harmful ingredients.

There are reasons to eat healthier, even though it may seem like it takes a harder hit on your wallet. If you can be more diligent in choosing more nutritious foods that keep you full longer, you won't have to buy as much food. For example, that big bag of chips is less expensive than the bag of apples, but you are more likely to go through the bag in one or two sittings where the bag of apples will last you closer to a week. Especially if you use your imagination and get creative. Spread some nut butter on that apple or add it to your oatmeal in the morning.

The fact is that the more sugar you eat, the more you crave it, and the more you are prone to overeat. If you make healthier choices that will help you to purchase less food and when you are not craving it as much and you are satisfying yourself by having smaller portions, you will be spending less. Eventually, the cravings for sugary items will subside, and there will not be a need to purchase them as often.

There are other ways to help your wallet when you are trying to eat healthier. Try to buy your produce seasonally and work your recipes around the fruits and vegetables that are lower in price. Keep an eye on your local flyers and make sure to find out what proteins are on sale that week as well. If you are more focused on taking care of yourself by eating healthy, you will more likely have fewer trips to the doctor and could save a lot of money by not having to take any medications or pay for prescriptions. In the long run, the excuses will run out, and eating healthy will be your best bet.

Don't let one more thing like the cost of healthy food be added to your list of things to stress out over. One of the leading causes that affect everyone at some point in their lives, some a lot more often than others, is stress.

Stress

Often the leading cause of emotional eating, about 40% of people tend to eat more when stressed, while about 40% eat less and 20% experience no change in the amount of food they eat when exposed to stress (Dryden-Edwards, 2017). There's a biological connection between emotional eating and stress, and that is because your body starts producing a hormone called cortisol when you start feeling alarmed or upset. This naturally occurring cortisol makes us crave those sugary, salty, addictive snacks. The more uncontrolled stress you have in your life, the more you turn to food to help feel in control. When stress is high, turning to our favorite treat makes us feel better by rewarding our pleasure center in the brain, but since it is short lived, you might keep it going by eating more or more often throughout the day. When extra weight is gained, the stress from feeling guilty and unattractive piles on along with the extra pounds. It is another vicious cycle, difficult to overcome.

The best way to stop yourself from eating when you are stressed is to try and deal with stress in other, more productive and positive ways. Writing in a journal, meditating, yoga, and doing a calming activity among other things can help deal with your daily stress.

Keep yourself moving in other ways by going for walks, working out, or other activities you may enjoy that keep your body moving. Many studies have proved mindful meditation can aid in treatment for binge eating or emotional eating. Deep breathing exercises are simple to do at home or anywhere you find convenient.

Past Traumas

Situations that happened in our past that were traumatic stay with us our entire lives. Everyone handles them differently. Most of the time, the trauma (which leads to PTSD) comes first, and the binge eating comes later. About one in four people who binge eat have PTSD (Brody, 2015). Researchers think people binge eat to 'escape' the painful memories related to the traumatic event. Many researchers have reported a link between binging and post-traumatic stress disorder, which can happen after you've seen or gone through a violent or life-threatening event; PTSD is also related to problems with stress hormones and mood-boosting brain chemicals. Some examples are

- Physical or sexual abuse or assault
- Experiencing a life-threatening accident
- The violent or accidental death of a loved one
- Witnessing or experiencing terrorism or war
- Witnessing a heinous crime such as a murder or rape

When struggling with past traumas, individuals usually don't think much about anything else or are so preoccupied with their thoughts, the idea of planning their meals is probably neglected. By the time they realize they are hungry, they are starving and tend to overeat.

Depression and Low Self-Esteem

Depression and overeating can somewhat coincide as well. If overeating leads to weight gain and an inability to control binge eating, depression is likely to follow. Depression itself may also trigger overeating as a coping mechanism. Feeling sad is a major reason why people emotionally eat. You have seen the scenario many times as a funny situation on TV; a woman is upset over a breakup, and the first thing she wants to do is run to the freezer and annihilate a pint of ice cream. She doesn't even need the bowl, knowing she plans on finishing the tub.

Eating makes some people feel happy, at that moment. Our brain remembers when we enjoy something, and it triggers the dopamine reaction. Our brain will constantly want that feeling again, and just like a drug, we become addicted. Food can be used to temporarily silence your feelings, and by numbing yourself, you avoid the real issues at hand. There was even a study recently that found the happiest moments of a typical participant's day were the ones where he or she was eating something (Carnell, 2011). It's because it all circles back to the fact that eating foods high in fat, salt, or sugar releases feel-good hormones like dopamine, which activate pleasure centers in your brain.

When it comes to low self-esteem, this can be a bit of a vicious cycle. You have low self-esteem, so you eat your feelings, and that leads to weight gain, and your self-esteem suffers even more because you are unhappy with your outward appearance. You may have gained weight or developed some health problems related to eating unhealthy food, such as diabetes.

Boredom and Reward

We've all done it. Sitting at home, bored, and we open the fridge even though we probably know the items inside. Then we search through the pantry, not certain if we are hungry or just bored. A piece of fruit won't do, but you want something in the ballpark of sweet, salty, and all-around not very good for you. Maybe we are sitting around the house bored, or maybe we have something we need to be doing, like homework or chores, and we are procrastinating.

Everyone is different in what they find boring. So whatever reason we have for boredom, why do we end up heading to the snack fridge or the pantry full of chips and treats? When you are bored, the feelings that go along with that are generally negative. You don't feel happy, more annoyed, angry, or even anxious. So you reach for the unhealthy snack or eat all your goodies until you are bursting. You may have felt good for a short period, but it won't last, and you will probably end up feeling worse than you did before you were bored and chose to overeat.

Rewarding ourselves or others with food is a long-time tradition of many. You nailed that important client you have been after for months, you finished writing a book you have been working on for a year, or your son or daughter won the big game. These are all different scenarios where we think it's acceptable to reward ourselves with an indulgent dinner out of our favorite dish made at home. Social influences can play a role too when you get together with family or friends to dine out. Or if you feel the pressure to socialize, maybe you end up overeating.

Is Emotional Eating Bad?

When does this start to become a real problem? It is not necessarily a bad thing if you have done something that deserves a special night out at your favorite restaurant. You should be able to enjoy food, and you shouldn't feel guilty after every time you eat. Some experts will say that it is okay to emotionally eat once in a while: to eat for comfort, to celebrate, or for no particular reason but that you just want to. Sometimes just what you need is in your fridge or cupboards. Going to the gym or taking a walk isn't going to make you feel better this time, and you just want that piece of cake in the fridge that you've been saving. Frequently turning to food to mask your emotions or make yourself feel better is not healthy in the long run. You know your body and mind the best, and you know when it is becoming an issue. It's the way you handle—and regulate—your eating that makes the difference between a pleasurable endeavor and a real health concern.

Whether it's psychological or physiological, it's clear that foods have a powerful effect on our moods. When your emotions are causing you to overeat or turn to food, and you can't control it, you should consider it more of a problem that you can take the time to dissect and come up with why you are using food to cope.

Why is emotional eating talked about like it's a bad thing? Maybe it's effective at the moment? Maybe it's the restricting part that you are reacting to? Yes, relying too much on food for comfort can indeed, in certain cases, be a problem for someone. If food is the only thing that you turn to in order to deal with uncomfortable feelings, that is a problem. It's true that food isn't meant to just be fuel. It's central to celebration, social bonding, tradition, happiness, and more, and it has been for centuries. The occasional celebration with friends at a restaurant or eating a cookie when you weren't hungry, you just wanted it, shouldn't be overthought. Maybe you are too strict with your intake, maybe you are overthinking, or maybe you need a better understanding of the difference between physical hunger and emotional hunger.

Chapter 3: Physical Hunger vs. Emotional Hunger

Know that emotional eating is normal and so many people use food as a coping mechanism or a way to be social. A lot of people struggle with knowing if they are hungry or eating for other reasons like stress, mood, or other emotions. Based on mindful eating, there are seven different types of hunger, all related to different organs of our body: mind, heart, eyes, nose, mouth, cells, and stomach. It is said that once a person gets aware of all these different types of hunger, one can make a healthy and conscious choice of what to eat and when. You might struggle more if you are a chronic dieter or often restrict foods from your diet. Whatever the reason you struggle, it is important to know the difference between physical hunger and emotional hunger because there is a big difference.

Physical hunger: Stomach grumbling, feeling weak or lethargic, low blood sugar, and lightheadedness are some of the common signs of physical hunger.

- You can instinctually tell when you are hungry
- Comes on slow and can usually wait if needed
- You know when you are full and can stop once you are full
- You feel satisfied without any guilt
- You can satisfy your hunger while still enjoying your food
- You understand your body's need for nutrition
- If you are full, you can leave food on the plate
- You are open to different meal options
- No negative feelings about food

Emotional hunger: As you have learned already, emotional hunger can't be satisfied with food. It might temporarily feel good, but the feelings that triggered the eating will remain and will only keep you in the cycle of emotional eating. Emotional hunger can be powerful, so it's easy to mistake it for physical hunger.

- Comes on suddenly
- Feels like it needs instant satisfaction
- Craving for specific comfort foods, usually unhealthy, high calorie, or processed
- Having a full stomach doesn't satisfy you
- Feelings of guilt, shame, and regret are triggered after eating
- You feel like you have no control
- Food suggestions or mentions of food in conversations might trigger you to want food
- Your desire to eat increases with certain emotions (stress, boredom, sadness, etc.)
- You eat mindlessly and don't realize how much you've eaten until you are uncomfortably full

- No matter how full you get, you never feel satisfied

When you know the difference between physical and emotional eating, you are able to be much more mindful of your habits when it comes to hunger and food. The more you are aware of why you are eating, the better. Knowing whether or not it is because you are physically hungry or feeling a certain emotional way can be beneficial to your success.

How Our Ancestors Treated Food and Eating

Thinking all the way back to the Stone Age, cavemen used to hunt for food and cook their game on hot stones or over a fire with no refrigerator and no real way to keep their food preserved. Fast forward to today, and there is a lot that has changed when it comes to the quality of your food. It is certainly nothing like what it was like when cavemen walked the earth! Cavemen had to work a lot harder for their food compared to the way it is now. Walking into the grocery store and picking out our packaged foods, including meat is much more convenient. There is even a section in some supermarkets where you can pick out a live lobster and take it home to cook yourself. Much easier than hunting, gathering, and foraging like the cavemen did.

What has changed so drastically over the years that we treat and eat food so differently? The advances in technology each year are incredible, but has society changed drastically to follow? Our ancestors certainly didn't have to deal with sugar addictions and carb loading. Cavemen were omnivorous; they loved plants and roots along with eating berries and seeds. They also fed on what they were able to hunt and fish because they did what they had to do to fill their bellies. Cooking was over a fire or on hot stones, and much of their food was consumed raw. As humans have evolved, meat has become more of the star of the show. Eating meat started to become essential as humans needed more energy, and they weren't getting enough from plants. It was said to have been able to fuel our larger growing brains.

The human body has had to adapt and change to adjust to the different sources of food that become abundant through time. The agriculture boom saw more wheat, grains, and beans being harvested as an abundant food source. With a longer shelf life and more convenience than the small window, you had to enjoy foods like fresh fruit. Wheat and beans became the primary food source, and even though it was critical for survival when other sources became scarce, they did bring other health concerns to the table.

Struggling to survive in an environment that offered few options between feast and famine, humankind could now grow its food. Farmers held livestock for meat and dairy, and we had more variety of foods to eat. It has been pondered whether agriculture was a step forward for human health, or, in leaving behind the hunter-gatherer ways to grow crops and raise livestock, was a healthier diet and stronger bodies given up in exchange for food security? Diets became less nutritional, Eating the same domesticated grain every day gave early farmers cavities, iron deficiency, and developmental delays. Even though the population was able to rise, this new diet even brought new infectious diseases.

Humans evolved from a vegetarian diet, and the digestive structures weren't especially adapted to eating meat. That is why it is beneficial to eat a fiber-rich vegetable source or salad and carbs like bread along with your main meat dish for better digestion. Cavemen didn't have access to the kind of preservatives available nowadays that increase shelf life for months or longer.

It's not too far-fetched to think of eating like cavemen. After all, the paleo diet is based on the way men ate before the wheel was invented. Paleo believers say since our genetics and anatomy haven't changed much since the Stone Age, we should eat foods available during that time to promote good health. Humans evolved in the wild where food was hard to come by, so if we did find a source of high-calorie foods, eating as much of it as possible would provide us with valuable stores for more scarce periods ahead. Humans will always continue to evolve, and it has been said that a Stone Age diet is a diet that ideally fits the human genetic makeup.

The biggest change that has happened to understand how humans are evolving is lactose tolerance. When cows started to be domesticated, and children were weaned off mother's milk, humans stopped making the enzyme lactase, which breaks down the lactose into simple sugars. It was harder for those unable to properly digest milk and often meant having to cut it out of their diet or suffer painful stomach issues. Cultures that did not use cows as a main food source actually were able to stay lactose tolerant.

Diabetes was virtually unknown until high sugar processing was introduced to the diet. Much of the weight gain that is becoming more prominent today is due to the fact that your food is cooked. There are a couple of ways we can increase our calories and cause our food to become less nutritious. One way is cooking out the nutrients with frying, boiling, and grilling your food in copious amounts of butter. Back when cavemen ate their food raw, it was actually the most nutritious way to prepare food, but things have obviously changed over time. Now humans are receiving more calories than they are burning, and that is where obesity and other health concerns start to come up.

Early humans figured out their own way to preserve their game, not wanting to waste what they worked so hard to hunt and kill. Salting, smoking, and drying are preservation techniques used for thousands of years. Sun-drying was a dominant food preservation method during the prehistoric period. Items were left in the sunshine to dry, but they weren't able to maintain longevity. Fruits were dried much of the time, and that is a process still used today. Preserving fruit by drying or turning into jams is a great way not to waste foods that easily spoil over time. Curing was another good way to preserve food by using a natural ingredient like salt. The brine was effective in killing bacteria. Later down the road, it was discovered that canning and pasteurization worked well in the ways of preserving.

Sugar was a natural preservative and could be combined with other preserving methods. Sugar has also, unfortunately, led to many issues today with overconsumption, weight gain, and health conditions such as diabetes. Before the 19th century, being thick was admired and meant you were wealthy, receiving an abundance of food. Heading into the 19th and 20th centuries, it was realized the long-term health effects that came with weight gain and obesity. Eventually, technological advances provided more knowledge, and preservatives started to evolve and become much better, and it was easier to have products with a longer shelf life. Refrigerators came around, and that was a game changer. Dehydration was a method used frequently, as well as vacuum sealing,

Today, we are able to go online, take approximately 10 minutes or so out of our day, and choose our weekly grocery list. We then pay a small fee, and someone can deliver it right to your doorstep! So you see how much food and eating habits have changed up until the present day. Much could change in the way of healthy eating to make sure disease or obesity doesn't progress.

Processed foods and chemicals are what humans have to live with today. Now, food manufacturers use additives to make a low-quality product look and taste great. Many of the foods on the shelves today have some degree of processing, but chemically processed foods tend to be high in sugar, artificial ingredients, refined carbohydrates, and trans fats. These foods also contain less dietary fiber and fewer vitamins than whole foods. Many countries regulate the use of chemicals in food, but that does not mean you should not still avoid these types of food when you can or only use them in moderation. Most of the items at fast-food chains are difficult for the body to digest, and that goes the same for highly processed foods on the grocery shelves. Other chemicals you might use or consume daily can include the following:

- **Herbicides and pesticides:** The adverse health effects harm the body, can lead to soil pollution, and the genetics of plants may get altered.
- **Preservatives:** Chemicals such as potassium sorbate may be harmful to us. Nitrites, a preservative in processed meats, may raise your cancer risk, and sodium benzoate, a common food additive, may cause hyperactivity

in children. Another popular preservative, sodium nitrite is a known carcinogen.

- **Food enhancers:** MSG is used in many foods to flavor them. MSG is an excitotoxin, which means it over-excites your cells. Excitotoxins can also kill or damage your brain cells. MSG can also cause breathing problems, headaches, numbness, and drowsiness among other side effects.

- **Food coloring:** These are used in certain drinks, candy, and ice cream. They can lead to hyperactivity in children, cancer, and allergies.

- **Artificial sweeteners:** These can cause you to overeat, and overconsumption can lead to intestinal gas, cramps, and diarrhea if you overeat them. Aspartame is one of the most dangerous and can lead to a wide variety of ailments such as ADD, brain tumors, diabetes, arthritis, and the list goes on.

If you are moody, tired, foggy, or irritable for unknown reasons, you are probably eating too many processed foods. Other symptoms can be feeling thirsty and bloated all the time, headaches, cavities, or tooth decay. Some other effects could be your hair could be thinning, and the big one is you aren't losing weight. All reasons could add up to the number of preservatives and prepackaged dinners you are consuming.

Even though humans have somewhat evolved through the years, that doesn't change the fact that our bodies are still the same as when we were cavemen. It is best to eat food in its natural state, eat what nature created, and not what humans manufactured. The more whole and natural a food is, the better. Try to grab an orange or an apple instead of turning to the juice form. Frozen, prepared meals are some of the worst things you can put in your body. It is much more beneficial to try and cook at home and from scratch. Even your soups can easily be made from scratch in large quantities and frozen for later meals. Keep low sodium broth, broth cubes, or powdered broths on hand. All good steps to having a healthier diet.

The Seven Types of Hunger

Being aware of these types of pangs of hunger gives us a better awareness and understanding of how to satisfy them. Our senses are activated by food, and these 'hungers' occur as sensations, thoughts, and even emotions within our bodies, minds, and hearts. It is easy to be fooled by our senses telling us we are hungry, even if we aren't. Here are the seven types of hunger that attempt to urge us to eat:

1. **Eye hunger:** You are reading through a magazine, and the advertisement has strategically placed a larger-than-it-looks cheeseburger on the page. You can see the details of the juices in the patty, the water beads off the tomato, and the cheese melted perfectly in between. Your eyes have the power to convince your brain to override the signals from your stomach. That's why you might see a lot of restaurants use pictures in their menu to try and entice you to order that item, especially dessert. Dessert is most often ordered, even if you know you are full, because it looks so good that you can't say no.

2. **Nose hunger:** Imagine when you and a friend decide to catch a movie. You walk into the lobby and head to the booth to purchase your ticket. A wave of delicious-smelling popcorn

hits you, and by the time your debit card has approved the purchase for the movie, you are running to the concession stand for some hot, buttery popcorn even though you aren't even hungry. Everyone knows popcorn is part of the whole movie experience.

3. **Mouth hunger:** This is the mouth's desire for more sensations, if our foods can be crunchier, cheesier, creamier. This includes how sweet or salty we want our food and can depend on how we were brought up or our past traditions, etc. That is what advertisers focus on to draw you in, especially when they are trying to remind you how good your favorite food was and how much better it is now.

4. **Stomach hunger:** You may think your stomach tells you when you're hungry, but you know now that it is actually your brain that

tells you. Your tummy might rumble, and you think you are hungry, but hunger cues are self-taught, and it takes practice to sense when a grumbling stomach means actual hunger. Your stomach does get full, and you should know when you feel full, that you don't require any more food. Try to stop eating when your stomach is comfortably full.

5. **Cellular hunger:** One of the hardest hungers to sense, even though it's the original reason for eating. It goes back to yourself as a baby, instinctively knowing when you were hungry and when you were full. Even when you were a bit older or still a young child, you knew what your body needed to be full, and when you were thirsty, you knew you needed liquids. As you age, different sources may interrupt those cues, and we lose the instinctive ability.

6. **Mind hunger:** The mind can be difficult to satisfy and pick up on natural cues. We are deafened by our inner voice telling us that one type of food is better than another. Once a craving is satisfied, the mind will move on to the next thing to focus on. This hunger can be influenced by what we read, hear, and see. Some people can rely on internal cues, and others base it on what their minds tell them about meal times.

7. **Heart hunger:** Think of the times when food comforted you; your mom made you homemade soup when you weren't feeling good, or your grandma came to visit and baked your favorite pie. Some people eat trying to fill an empty hole in their hearts. This is the 'heart' of emotional eating. Your food is linked to your

emotions. That is why it is important to consider how you are feeling before you snack.

Next time you are hungry, try and figure out which of these senses you might be feeling or if you are just hungry. Try to be mindful of what and how you eat, take in the aroma, feast with your eyes, and savor every flavor. Don't rush through your food or have too many distractions. Only then will you be truly satisfied.

Chapter 4: How Do Hormones Play a Role?

It's important to know that losing weight or gaining it isn't all about calories and willpower; hormones can play a role in how your body responds to certain things and can be working against you. Keep in mind what the important hormones do when it comes to how our bodies respond to certain hormones, and how our bodies take in calories, the hormones in relation to the fat in our bodies, or how much or little we need of certain hormones.

Going back to our junior high science class, hormones are molecules that have the power to affect changes in our cells. You have tons of different hormones produced in your body for different functions, and your body is constantly sending messages to regulate these hormones in your body. Hormones can affect individuals in different ways. It is said that certain hormones that arrive during women's menstrual periods can have something to do with emotional eating. There are hormones that affect hunger, and that can play a role in your eating habits or the way your body changes or reacts.

How do hormones affect our emotions? Our emotions can change based on our hormones, just like our physical bodies can change. Hormones can be very powerful with only a small amount needed to create big changes. This is why our mood swings can feel so drastic when our hormones are out of balance. You need to understand that besides emotions, other powerful biological forces are causing you to indulge. Certain hormones play a role in this. For example, when you haven't eaten for a while, ghrelin levels increase. Then, after you've eaten, leptin levels tell your body that it's full. Your body needs a good balance of hormones to stay healthy; however, overeating may disrupt this balance. It's important to understand that you have a great deal of control over your hormones as they will always respond to the dietary and stress-related changes we make along with our exercise.

Ghrelin

Ghrelin has come to be known as the "hunger hormone" because it regulates your hunger and plays a role in controlling your appetite. Ghrelin is produced in the stomach and small intestine with a small amount of the hormone released in the pancreas and brain. It works to increase or decrease our appetite. It appears to help control insulin release and plays a protective role in cardiovascular health. Ghrelin is secreted by an empty stomach. Once you eat and stretch your stomach, the hormone will stop being secreted. Ghrelin aids in digesting more food and storing more fat; it is much more than a hunger hormone though. As a peptide hormone, it's produced by cells located in the gastrointestinal tract, which communicate with the central nervous system, especially the brain. Once produced in the stomach, the cells send a response to the brain that causes you to feel hungry.

There can be problems that follow the hormone. When those who suffer from certain eating disorders, such as anorexia nervosa, the levels of ghrelin are high because the body naturally produces it when dealing with starvation. Furthermore, when you are attempting to diet and restrict calorie intake, your body will also produce high levels of ghrelin. This hormone is also what gives you that snack attack and leads to the potential to overeat. It is also released directly to the brain when we feel stressed, and that is why many people turn to food when they are feeling particularly stressed out.

If you want ghrelin to work in your favor, there are a few things you should consider:

- **Don't restrict your calories too much:** Just like overeating decreases ghrelin, reducing your calories drastically will increase the hormone, and that isn't good for your body. Feeling hungry is the worst part of lowering your calories per day, but you can choose the proper foods to keep you feeling full. Eating plenty of healthy food will keep your body feeling more active and stop you from entering "starvation mode," which only makes your appetite that much stronger.
- **Eat enough protein:** Protein is a key staple food to help control your appetite. Protein

tends to keep you more satisfied longer, helps obtain muscle mass, helps with digestion, and improves your overall stability.

- **Stay away from highly processed food and empty calories:** They won't satisfy your hunger and will only increase your calorie count for the day. When we eat our food, normally a signal will enter our brain to tell us when we are full. When we consume highly processed foods, the feedback doesn't always get sent to the brain properly and interferes with appetite regulation.
- **Adequate sleep:** Lack of sleep or poor-quality sleep can disturb your levels of ghrelin and leptin, possibly intensifying food cravings, especially in the evenings, including the effects that sleep deprivation has on melatonin

production, and then ghrelin and leptin production.

- **Exercise often:** Exercising along with reducing stress, which has been mentioned, are all crucial to reducing the ghrelin effect of always feeling hungry.

The same area of the brain that holds the receptors for ghrelin is another hormone called leptin.

Leptin

Often referred to as the "satiety hormone" or the "starvation hormone," leptin is one of the hormones directly connected to body fat and obesity. It is released from the fat cells of adipose tissue in the body and sent to the brain. Leptin's main role is long-term regulation of energy, including the number of calories you eat and expend, as well as how much fat you store in your body. Since leptin comes from fat cells, the amount comes from the fat you have stored in your body; the more body fat you have, the more leptin you have, and, in turn, if you lose body fat, the leptin will decrease, and low levels tell your brain that fat stores are low and that you need to eat.

Leptin helps to regulate and alter the food you eat in the long term and aids with the amount of energy you expend, not just from one meal to the next. The primary design of leptin is to help the body maintain its weight. It helps inhibit hunger and regulate energy balance, so the body does not trigger hunger responses when it does not require energy. When you lose weight, the levels will fall, and this is what causes an increase in appetite, a spike in cravings, and hunger pangs. That is why it's so difficult to shed any weight you have been trying to.

There is such a thing as leptin resistance. In people who are considered obese, their brain should naturally be telling them they are full, and they should be limiting their food based on the high amount of body fat they maintain, but their signal for leptin may not be working. This resistance is known to be one of the main causes of obesity today. If your brain isn't properly receiving the signal, then you will continually overeat, thinking you are hungry. This is also a contributing factor in struggling to lose weight and keeping it off long term.

Again, diet, exercise, and sleep habits all play a part in reversing leptin resistance, and it would also help if you could lower your triglycerides, which is a type of fat found in your blood. Having high triglycerides can prevent the transport of leptin from your blood to your brain. The best way to lower triglycerides is to reduce how many carbohydrates you are eating in your diet.

Insulin

Insulin is produced and stored in the pancreas. If you are constantly eating, you are constantly producing insulin, one of the most misunderstood hormones. Too much insulin in your body can cause weight gain, and too little of it will cause serious health problems. When you eat starches, sugars, and other carbohydrates, they're digested into simple sugars in the intestine and are then released into the bloodstream. Insulin is in charge of signaling the muscle to absorb sugar, which is why we can't consume too much sugar and carbs since the insulin won't be able to keep up. The overload of sugar causes your body to frantically try to produce more insulin to keep levels consistent. That is also why, after consuming a lot of sugary treats, you experience that 'crash.' Blood sugar decreases and lowers your energy. Insulin stores any sugars you don't use for later, and eating too many carbs and not burning them throughout the day causes the production of fat in fat cells.

With consistent overeating of carbs, your cells start to ignore the insulin. For those who suffer from diabetes, their blood sugar levels are too high and don't produce enough insulin. With type 1 diabetes, your body cannot make insulin properly, and with type 2 diabetes, your body has become resistant to the effects of insulin. Insulin can be taken through a shot or a pump. With insulin helping maintain your blood sugar levels, you can function at your best.

Peptide YY

Are there different ways your body can recognize when you have eaten enough food? After eating, the hormone peptide YY (PYY) is produced by the small intestine and released into your bloodstream. PYY communicates to your brain that you are full and decreases your appetite. The amount of PYY released depends on the type of food you have eaten and how much. After it is released into your bloodstream, PYY attaches to the cells that receive signals in the brain. It also works by slowing down the movement of food in the digestive tract. Fat and protein are foods that especially produce PYY along with higher calorie foods. If large amounts of time go by without eating, your levels will go down.

The problem with PYY is that very high levels will decrease your appetite, and low levels will lead to weight gain. Having abnormal levels is rare, but it is important to know they could have something to do with your weight. Keeping your calories moderate and watching what you eat, of course, can help in keeping your levels normal, like some of the other hormones mentioned.

Cortisol

Cortisol is also known as the "stress hormone" and acts naturally in response to stress. Produced by the adrenal glands, cortisol has several functions other than just responding to stress. It assists in regulating your blood pressure, aids in glucose metabolism, immune function, inflammatory response, and helps with releasing insulin.

When we experience a stressful situation, cortisol is released. This process is also referred to as the "fight or flight" response, which is how our bodies respond to any situations that make you feel you are in danger or that your life is threatened. Your body prepares to either stay or leave the situation.

Of course, like anything, too much cortisol is not good for your health. Chronic stress from prolonged stress can cause a higher level of cortisol, which can lead to high blood pressure, blood sugar imbalance, lowered immunity, and other harmful effects. With higher cortisol and more body fat, specifically in the stomach area, there is more risk to your health, such as higher bad cholesterol and lower good cholesterol, increased risk for heart attacks, strokes, and metabolic syndrome.

Keep your stress levels low by practicing stress management methods to keep you more relaxed in body and mind. Meditation, journaling, yoga, breathing exercises, or other soothing activities that you find to suit your needs are best.

Estrogen and Progesterone

Estrogen and progesterone are sex hormones that women have. While it is responsible for the reproductive development of a woman, it can affect their emotions more during certain times in their everyday life. Both high and low levels can affect weight gain. For example, the menstrual period has a lot to do with food cravings and wanting something comforting that is more likely high in sugar, salt, and fat. Research has said that during the second half of your cycle, which spans from the day after ovulation to the day before your next period, you're two to four times more likely to turn to emotional eating than you are during the first half of your cycle (Lichterman, 2017).

Research has found that these two hormones affect you in two different ways throughout your menstrual cycle: During the first half of your cycle, while you're less likely to use food for comfort, when you do, it's because rising estrogen is making you more sensitive to certain situations in your environment. Other people or activities may influence your choices as well. During the second half of your cycle, which is a time when you're more prone to emotional eating, it's because progesterone is messing with your hormones and changes your mood, which leads to a better chance of turning to food to make your stress go away or make you feel better. Your urge to eat is much stronger during this time.

Another change in women, menopause, can also play a role in how women feel emotionally. There is less progesterone in women after experiencing menopause, and estrogen will drop as well. What about when a woman is pregnant? Progesterone spikes following the release of an egg from the ovary. It helps your body prepare for pregnancy after ovulation.

Ways to Fix the Hormones that Control Your Weight

There is no doubt hormones control our bodies in many different ways, and you know how many hormones control our weight, whether we have too much or too little of them. Here are some ways we can try to fix the hormones that we know have such control over your weight.

1. **Minimize your sugar intake:** You can't expect yourself to completely give up sugar cold turkey, but you can start to minimize your

intake and learn which foods have more sugar in them than you thought. Doctors say you shouldn't have more than six teaspoons, which is about 25 grams per day.

2. **Reduce carbs and fill up on protein:** If you want to lower your insulin, consume fewer carbs. Protein helps to raise insulin and reduce ghrelin, which, over a lengthy period, can help you lose belly fat.

3. **Have plenty of healthy fats in your diet:** Healthy fats in your diet, like omega-3, can help lower your insulin. Fish have plenty of omega-3 fats. Avocados are another healthy fat food that is easy to include in your salads, sliced on top of a bowl of chili, or spread over your toast.

4. **Make sure you get enough magnesium:** You can get magnesium supplements, and if

you are insulin-sensitive, that will help. Green vegetables like kale and spinach also provide a good amount of magnesium.

5. **Drink green tea:** Green tea has been known to lower blood sugar and insulin levels.
6. **Avoid inflammatory foods:** Limit foods that cause inflammation, especially sugary drinks and trans fats.
7. **Exercise regularly:** Of course, regular exercise can help with hormone sensitivity and normalize levels of hormones.

The key to balancing hormones naturally is to adopt some pretty basic, easy, but super important rules of healthy living. It can be as simple as having a healthy diet, exercising regularly, and reducing stress. Fortunately, diet and lifestyle changes can have powerful effects on these hormones.

Chapter 5: Importance of Diet and Exercise

It is not against the law to indulge every once in a while. It's best to enjoy high-calorie snacks in moderation and stay regular with a healthy diet and exercise. Diet and exercise go hand-in-hand and are important to focus on to stay healthy and live a longer, happier life. Some may think that you can indulge in any foods you want as long as you exercise enough, but that is not the case in terms of a healthy lifestyle long term.

It's not about jumping on the new diet bandwagon but changing your lifestyle goals to continue with new, positive habits. With a new and popular fad diet hitting the streets all too often, not to mention what was healthy yesterday could be the opposite the next day, how are you supposed to keep up? That is why you are much better off with a true lifestyle change that includes making lifelong changes and better routines, not a quick fix diet that gains you five extra pounds as soon as you move on. It might seem like quite a feat now, but, depending on your determination, it only takes about 18 days to form a habit, and in no time, you can have some health goals for the long term.

It is important to start small, making small changes for longer-lasting effects. If you change everything too quickly, you are more likely to crash and burn. Don't be afraid to take baby steps. Here are some easy, small steps to get you going in the right direction:

- Start by adding at least one serving of fruit or vegetables to every meal and even switch your snacks to include them. Be a little sneaky by adding finely grated carrots or zucchini to pasta sauce, meatloaf, chili, or a stew to get in that extra serving of vegetables.

- Replace the soda you drink every day with club soda. Drinking too many sugary sodas can increase your desire for high-calorie foods and put you at risk for weight gain. Club soda will still give you the bubbles you might crave. Freeze some sliced strawberries and add to your water for some natural flavor.

- Take the stairs every opportunity you can. Soon it will just become a habit to skip the elevator.

- Instead of using too much salt on your food or recipes, try using more spices and fresh herbs. Adding flavor that way makes a difference and lessens your sodium intake.

- Keep more healthy items at home and rearrange your cupboards so your healthy staples are always within sight and within reach.

- Start with a 10 minute walk in the morning, after dinner, or try to devote some of your lunch break to a quick walk. Each week, try to increase this time by 5 to 10 minutes until you can reach an hour. Eventually try to incorporate some time to a more brisk walk every day, until eventually you can make it more intense. Even getting outside as often as you can is good for your mood, and just 20 minutes in the sun gives you the vitamin D you need for the day.

Eating healthy is important, and being able to make more of your meals at home is best because you know what ingredients are going in, and you can control the amount of salt you use in your recipes. When you eat out, you have no clue how much salt, butter, or oil is going into your meal, not to mention the portion sizes are probably too much. When you cook meals for yourself at home, make sure you cook another portion so you can take your healthy leftovers to work or school. You are much less likely to go for a fast food run during lunch when you know you have your lunch set out for you every day.

Beware of healthy food items that may seem like they are a better choice. Take-out or dine-in restaurants that claim to be healthy have all kinds of hidden preservatives and highly processed foods. Certain "fat-free" foods are probably higher in things like sodium. Granola bars might seem like a good choice, but they are actually high in sugar and not very filling. If you think a salad is a healthy choice, you are right, but be aware of creamy dressing and certain toppings that can add calories. Even your protein could be unhealthy if it's breaded chicken instead of grilled.

Having a good habit of exercising regularly can contribute highly not only to your physical health but also to your mental health. Exercise releases endorphins that leave you feeling naturally euphoric and in a state of happiness. Working out for just 30 minutes a few times a week can instantly boost your overall mood. Regular exercise can have a greatly positive impact on stress, depression, anxiety, and ADHD. Exercise has proven to be an effective activity with positive outcomes for those who suffer from different mental illnesses.

When it comes to suffering from depression, exercise has been shown to promote all kinds of changes in the brain, including neural growth, reduced inflammation, and new activity patterns that promote feelings of calm and well-being. Working out can serve as a good distraction from the hub of the day-to-day. It could grow into something you look forward to doing by yourself or with someone you care about. Stress can take a toll on our bodies if it is prolonged. As you know, stress can have long-term effects and can be detrimental to your immune system. Exercising frequently can actually boost your immune system. Stress levels are lower in those who are frequent with their workouts, and physical activity helps to relax the muscles and relieve tension in the body. Exercise also helps with anxiety levels because it stabilizes your mood and decreases levels of tension. This also has an impact on those with ADHD because exercise improves your concentration, motivation, memory, and mood. Lastly, for those who suffer with PTSD and trauma, your body goes through positive changes when you workout, and you can help your nervous system to get out of your funk more and begin to move out of the immobilization stress response that characterizes PTSD or trauma. Being able to enjoy exercise outside or in nature is even more effective with those who suffer from a mental health disorder. Exercise can help you build resilience and cope with your mental health more constructively instead of resorting to destructive alternatives like alcohol, hard drugs, or other negative behaviors that ultimately only make your symptoms worse.

Exercise is a large part of maintaining a healthy lifestyle. It is not the right attitude to think you can eat whatever you want as long as you offset it with exercise. The problem with that thinking is an unhealthy diet does not include all the nutrients your body needs and often includes foods that are high in calories and low in nutrients. Moderate- to high-intensity cardio exercise strengthens the heart, allowing it to push more blood into your body with each heartbeat. Less stress on the heart means your risk of heart disease is lowered. Regular exercise may also help manage hunger by regulating your hunger hormones. This may help prevent overeating and excess snacking. Excessive exercise can also lead to increased appetite, so if you keep it in moderation, you are better off. Research has proven many times over that diet combined with exercise is best for overall health.

Strength training or resistance training uses weights to build endurance and stamina. It is good to add to your workout routine at least twice a week. Aerobic exercise or cardio is a more intense exercise that gets your heart rate going. That could be anything from brisk walking to swimming to biking.

There are many benefits to these types of exercise:

1. **Increases your bone density:** Inactive bones become active, and your strength training can decrease muscle spasms, bone

fractures, osteoporosis or osteoarthritis, and vitamin D deficiency.

2. **Keep your body fit over time:** Everyday activities can be much easier, like carrying groceries or playing with your kids. Your body will stay fit and in good shape.

3. **Boost your metabolism:** This helps your body to burn more calories. With resistance training, you continue to burn calories long after your workout.

4. **Keeps your heart and lungs healthy:** Your lungs inhale more oxygen with this exercise, which improves lung capacity but also blood circulation and heart health.

5. **Boosts brain power:** Your brain functions better, and research has proven better brain response and memory overall. With age, your brain starts to shrink. While exercise can't cure

Alzheimer's, it can help with cognitive decline as we age.

6. **Provides sufficient sleep:** Exercising five or six hours before bedtime raises your body's temperature, and when your temp drops back to normal a few hours later, it signals to your body that it's time to sleep. You will feel more relaxed and enjoy a better sleep overall.

7. **Increases your confidence:** The outcome of keeping up with your workouts is the boost in your positive self-image. Feeling good is bound to happen when you have more energy and your pants always fit!

Keeping a healthy lifestyle by including a consistently healthy diet and exercise is one of the best ways to prevent disease. It can help to prevent cardiovascular disease, certain cancers, type 2 diabetes, obesity, and even anxiety and depression. You will feel more energized.

Everyone is aware of the importance of a good breakfast. Why is that? Your breakfast is the first meal after you wake up, hopefully from an adequate seven to nine hours of sleep. This meal is going to fuel you for the rest of the morning, and if you have a busy schedule, it might be a while before you have a lunch break. If you reach for something you think is quick and easy, like cereal, the majority of them are loaded with sugars and refined grains. A better choice that you can easily squeeze into your morning routine would be oatmeal with berries and bananas. Instead of a doughnut or a croissant that will probably only keep you full for a short time and cause that sugar crash later in the day, go for more whole grains. Some whole or multigrain bread can be satiated by adding various proteins like nut butter, or you could easily spread on some avocado for a serving of healthy fats.

Overnight oats are easy to make the night before for an even quicker healthy breakfast on the go. They are a great source of fiber and protein, and you can switch them up with different items you happen to have in your fridge. They are a real time-saver since you prepare them ahead of time. All you need is oats, any type of milk including almond or oat milk, and berries.

Get creative by adding the following:

- Chia seeds
- Nut butter
- Yogurt
- Protein powder
- Granola
- Coconut

- Other fresh fruits

All you need to do is add the milk, yogurt, seeds, and bananas to a jar with a lid and refrigerate overnight. In the morning, add more liquid of your choice and additional toppings.

Carbs are not the enemy here. In fact, they are the opposite because they are your body's main source of energy. If you cut them completely out of your diet, once you re-introduce them, you could risk quick weight gain. Studies show, especially if you are combining exercise, about 45 to 65% of your total daily calories should come from carbohydrates (Rosenbloom, 2009). It is more beneficial to include complex carbs into your meals, which is part of a healthy, balanced diet. Some complex carbs include the following:

1. Vegetables like broccoli, potatoes, tomatoes, onions, carrots, yams, spinach, zucchini, cucumber, asparagus, radishes, or peas.
2. Fruits like strawberries, apples, pears, prunes, or grapefruit.
3. Whole grains like buckwheat, brown rice, wheat, barley, oats, corn, or quinoa.
4. Nuts, seeds, and legumes, like lentils, kidney beans, chickpeas, soybeans, pinto beans, or soy milk.

There are many benefits of including complex carbs in your diet:

- They provide fuel for your body for longer periods.
- They slow digestion, which makes you feel full longer.
- They aid in healthy weight loss by helping you control those urges to grab an unhealthy snack.

- They aid in heart health by lowering cholesterol and blood pressure.

When food is processed or refined, it's lacking most of its fiber, vitamins, and minerals, and often preservatives are added in their place. A diet that's low in these nutrients may cause you to feel hungry or experience cravings, even if you have otherwise eaten enough calories. That is why nutrients are so important to your diet.

The Importance of Nutrients

The best decision you can make is the decision to keep yourself healthy. By losing the fad diets and latest trends and sticking to a variety of the most nutrient-dense foods available—in other words, unprocessed, whole foods—will lead you to feel more satisfied and remain healthy. Nutrients are there to help you stay healthy, and there are nutrients to be aware of that aid in helping you feel more full. They are there to provide nourishment essential for growth and the maintenance of life. If you can eat more filling foods and lower your calories, you can stop that extra weight gain. Having a balanced diet helps to make sure you have a proper amount of nutrients in your diet. Nutrients like protein and fiber can help you feel full. If you are lacking important nutrients in your diet, it can lead to symptoms of possible nutritional deficiencies that can include both physical and mental symptoms such as

- Fatigue or confusion
- Dry skin
- Reduced immune function
- Dizziness
- Brain function

If you aren't sure if your diet has enough nutrients, here is a list of nutrient-rich foods:

- Avocados
- Chard, collard greens, kale, mustard greens, spinach
- Bell peppers
- Brussels sprouts
- Mushrooms (crimini and shiitake)
- Potatoes (white or sweet)
- Cantaloupe, papaya, raspberries, strawberries
- Yogurt
- Eggs—in just one 75 calorie egg, you'll get vitamin B, choline, vitamin D, plus healthy fats like omega-3, and some protein.
- Seeds (flax, pumpkin, sesame, sunflower)
- Beans (garbanzo, kidney, navy, pinto)
- Lentils, peas
- Almonds, cashews, peanuts

- Barley, oats, quinoa, brown rice
- Salmon, halibut, cod, scallops, shrimp, tuna
- Lean beef, lamb, venison
- Chicken, turkey

Be careful because there are ways you could be destroying the nutrients in your foods without even knowing it. Many factors can influence the nutrients in the foods we eat such as depleted soils, food manufacturing, processing and shipping, and even when we cook and heat them at home. According to research, broccoli, which is one of the superfoods we all know is good for us, has lost 63 percent of its calcium and 34 percent of its iron (Superfoods: Broccoli Benefits, Nutrition and You, 2015). Your best way to cook your vegetables, as not to lose more precious nutrients, would be to steam them. Boiling them in water is one of the top ways to lose nutrients.

Some other ways to keep the nutrients in your fruits and vegetables are

1. **Buy locally grown:** You have less time for shipping that depletes your nutrients with time.
2. **Start growing in your own garden:** What could be quicker than going to your backyard for the greens you need?
3. **Choose frozen over fresh more often:** Nutrients are locked in by being frozen immediately after harvest.
4. **Eat them in bigger pieces:** Don't chop your fruits and veggies too small; bigger pieces have less exposure to air and suffer less loss of nutrients.
5. **Washing:** Wash your fruit to remove pesticides, but don't soak them as this removes nutrients and water-soluble vitamins.

6. **Dehydrate your fruits and veggies:** Drying out your fruit is a good way to preserve the nutrients, and it makes a delicious, healthy snack such as pears, apples, apricots, pineapples, carrots, beetroot, and potatoes.

Fiber-rich foods are also essential for your health and are great at keeping you full and satisfied. Good sources include fruits, vegetables, whole grains, nuts, and, best of all, dark chocolate. Fiber goals are different depending on your age and gender. The recommended amounts are

- **Men ages 50 or younger:** 38 grams
- **Men over 50:** 30 grams
- **Women ages 50 or younger:** 25 grams
- **Women over 50:** 21 grams

Food is not meant to make you feel happy. You have to do that for yourself, but there are foods out there that can contribute to your mood. It has to do with the brain and how your mood is regulated.

You know the brain uses neurotransmitters as communication signals to tell your body certain commands, like breathing and your heart beating. When keeping your mood stable, your brain also uses neurotransmitters called excitatory neurotransmitters, like norepinephrine that stimulate our bodies and minds, and inhibitory neurotransmitters, like serotonin that calm down our minds. Our mood is the best when both of these neurotransmitters are balanced.

It is important to know that these neurotransmitters don't come out of anywhere. They can be created by compounds in the foods we eat. That is why there are such foods, happy foods that can help with your mood. Foods known to increase serotonin, which is the happy neurotransmitter, are turkey, spinach, and bananas. Spinach contains high concentrations of folate, a B-vitamin used in the serotonin creation process. Bananas and turkey have a high amount of tryptophan, an amino acid that's converted into serotonin in the brain. Very scientific but interesting to know what the food you eat can do to your mood. A healthy balance of nutritious foods and comfort foods can help maintain the balance in a person's mood best of all.

Everyone has foods that make them feel better, give them nostalgia, and bring them together with friends and family. Studies have shown that eating comfort food not only activates our brain's pleasure centers but also activates touch centers as well. Comfort foods are even enjoyed more when the weather is cold. Being cold is deeply uncomfortable, and our natural instinct is to want to warm ourselves both inside and out with food. Research has shown that personally defined "comfort foods" do improve mood after a stressful event, but they don't do a better job than any other foods. The idea that some foods are uniquely comforting is a cognitive illusion likely driven by the difficulty your brain has making rational decisions when under stress. These comfort foods are hard to give up.

When people are sad, they are more likely to indulge in comfort foods than when they are happy to improve their mood. What you think you want and what you actually want can be very different, and your brain has clever ways of tricking you into believing otherwise. Choosing satisfying foods that are both warm and nutritious is one strategy to break the spell of comfort foods. Another is to realize that food is only one form of comfort. If you know that something warm will make you feel better, maybe a warm tea or a hot bath will suffice. There are comfort foods out there that are healthy. They might need a bit of tweaking with less butter and salt and more vegetables incorporated.

Staying Hydrated

There are multiple health reasons to drink plenty of water. Doctors have always encouraged individuals to try and drink at least eight ounces of water a day, or two liters, but most recently, it is highly recommended to drink 11.5 cups for women and 15.5 cups for men. Every day, you lose water through your breath, perspiration, urine, and bowel movements, so it is important to replenish it throughout the day (Mayo Clinic, 2020b). Water helps to regulate your temperature, lubricates and cushions your joints, protects your spinal cord and other sensitive tissues, and gets rid of wastes through urination, sweat, and bowel movements. Since 50 to 75 percent of your weight is water, drinking some plain old H2O is imperative in keeping your body working the best it can and staying hydrated.

How much water can depend on some other factors as well:

1. **Where you live:** You will need more water in hot, humid, or dry areas. You'll also need more water if you live in the mountains or at a high altitude.
2. **Your diet:** If you drink a lot of coffee and other caffeinated beverages, you might lose more water through extra urination. If your diet is high in salty, spicy, or sugary foods, you will likely need to drink more water as well. More water is also necessary if you don't eat a lot of hydrating foods high in water like fresh or cooked fruits and vegetables.

3. **The temperature or season:** You may need more water in warmer months than cooler ones due to the heat and how much you sweat.

4. **Your environment:** If you spend more time outdoors in the Sun, hot temperatures, or a heated room, you might feel thirstier faster.

5. **How active you are:** If you are active during the day or walk or stand a lot, you'll need more water than someone who's sitting at a desk. If you exercise or do any intense activity, you will need to drink more to cover water loss.

Did you know if you feel hungry, you might just be thirsty? Before you head to the cupboards or fridge, try drinking a glass of water first. It is beneficial to be drinking plenty of water throughout the day. Drinking a full glass of cold water can help wake you up and boost your alertness first thing in the morning. It is especially beneficial to drink a full glass of tepid water with lemon first thing in the morning. The reasoning behind this is that it is a holistic practice said to soothe the digestive system, boost your immune system, and hydrate your lymphs.

There are a few ways you can try to increase your intake of water simply:

- Try drinking an extra glass of water each day until you are up to eight servings. Set realistic goals for yourself in achieving more intake each day until you are satisfied.
- Try carrying around a water bottle that has measurements to keep track of your intake. Leave it at your work desk, in the car, and anywhere as a reminder.
- Set alarms and reminders for yourself so you don't forget or get too busy with your day-to-day activities. There are apps out there to remind you as well.

- Flavor your water with fruits like lemon, strawberry, or add cucumber or mint. There are water enhancers out there, but just be aware of the sugar, fructose, or artificial sweetener content.
- Eat foods high in water. There are several foods that contain over 90% water, such as lettuce, celery, zucchini, cucumber, watermelon, cantaloupe, and honeydew.

Drinking water can cause slight, temporary increases in metabolism, and drinking it about a half-hour before each meal can help you eat fewer calories. There are so many benefits to something simple as water, not to mention the money you will save by not buying all those sugary drinks, but the most important benefit of drinking plenty of water overall, particularly before meals, is the boost you might get in managing appetite and maintaining a healthy body weight, especially when combined with a healthy eating plan.

Making It a Lifestyle Change

Try to start having a better relationship when it comes to food, not only being aware of when you emotionally eat but making sure you cultivate a more positive relationship. Instead of thinking about all the food you can't have or shouldn't include in your diet, try to incorporate all the foods you can eat and want to include that are healthy and delicious. There are foods out there that can make for a wonderful meal that is also good for you.

Every journey can look different and unique to every person. Perhaps you feel like you drink more than you would like, and that is deterring your goals. Most cocktails and beer are high in calories, so they can add up and end up increasing your calorie intake for the day. Something as simple as taking out alcohol for a while can help. You can start by cutting back and seeing how you feel. Generally, overconsumption of alcohol can make you tired and have less energy.

If you want to stick to your new lifestyle plan, make sure you have it well documented, and make yourself a plan of action to follow. Write out what you plan to have for healthy meals including your breakfast, lunch, dinner, and snacks. Write a separate list of what you will need from the grocery store for your weekly meal plan. Do not stray from your list, but you can have a couple of indulgence items as long as you write them into your plan and limit them to keep yourself on track. You don't want to deprive yourself completely, and everyone is entitled to a cheat day.

Documenting your new lifestyle includes meal plans and writing out what you have consumed every day from your morning coffee down to your after-dinner snack. If you can look back and see what exactly you are consuming, you can catch yourself when you might have a bad day or overindulge. You can ask yourself why that happened. What was different that day that made you change course? If you have any snack foods in your house that are too tempting for you at the start, you might think of donating them to a food bank or giving them to a friend. You don't need any unwanted distractions or anything that might make you break, especially when you first decide to make a change in your lifestyle.

A great way to keep your lifestyle goals is to figure out what stage you are at in your life to make sure you are at the proper stage to keep it going. You can't start a race at the finish line, can you? What stage of change are you in?

1. **Contemplation:** During this stage, you are thinking about all the positive lifestyle changes you want to make, and you are feeling motivated to pursue but haven't quite committed to following through. You are well aware you need to make some healthy changes in your life, but you might be afraid to start with anything too drastic. You are unsure how to get over some of the hurdles you are facing with the decision.

2. **Preparation:** This is the stage where you have decided to take action. You may be coming up with more specific ideas to put your changes into action. You have some goals written out to have them more top of mind, and you are

getting ready to move forward with your new lifestyle change.

3. **Action:** In this stage, you are taking action on your plan to make a new lifestyle change. The goals you have set out for yourself will be put into action. You might start to get rid of any snack in your house that can sway your goals, or you might go out and get a gym membership. You are starting small by getting better sleep and being more active. You have been taking steps to get over anything that might be blocking you from your goals.

4. **Maintenance:** The final stage, where now your plans are part of a new lifestyle and a new routine. You have gotten used to your new changes and even formed some new, positive habits. Your changes have become a normal part of your routine, and you don't have to

think too much about the new goals you have managed to meet. You have found creative ways to make your goals stick and have managed to get over all of your barriers that were tripping you up in the past or causing you to fear.

If you find you have a lot of reasons why you can't or won't start a lifestyle change, write them all down and come up with some solutions ahead of time. Write out a list of pros and cons to why you want to start working out or eating healthier. The chances of failing will be much less if you already have a plan and a list of solutions. If you have a setback, don't beat yourself up. It's bound to happen, you're only human, so just get back up and keep going. Go over your setbacks and solutions again. If you are doing exceptionally well with your goals, don't be afraid to adjust them a bit and challenge yourself a bit more, only if you are comfortable of course.

Don't be afraid to reward yourself for great accomplishments. That doesn't mean you have to give yourself a full cheat day and feel regretful after. This could include a day out at the spa or a little shopping spree. Maybe there is a new pair of yoga pants you have been eyeing, and you could buy them in a few months when you are a size down.

Whether or not losing weight is a high priority on your list of why you want a lifestyle change, there are always going to be hurdles and difficult challenges that will try to trip you up in your journey. Have you ever noticed how happy all the people are in commercials? Especially when they are eating a greasy hamburger? They seem to have it all and they look like people who would never have to worry about emotional eating. Right?

Chapter 6: The Effects of Advertising

The average American encounters 3,000 advertisements every day (Roeder, 2015b). What you see on TV, the internet, and especially social media can often be misleading. Food is available 24 hours a day, 7 days a week, and the food industry knows that and takes advantage of it to sell their products and turn a big profit. There are television shows that do the same thing as advertisers do. They make food look comforting and don't show the real problems it can cause for people long-term and the real issues behind suffering from emotional eating. It goes back to the time when products were advertised, and the information they provided was misleading. While outright lies are not allowed in advertising, lies of omission are common, and advertisements frequently prey on our emotions to get us to buy into what they are telling us. There was a time in advertising where people didn't even realize how much photoshop was being used. There are so many aspects of advertising we may be unaware of being used to sway us.

For example, products would say they were recommended by a doctor or dermatologist when the truth is those testimonials aren't actually regulated. The truth, when it comes to shopping for beauty products that claim "used most by dermatologists" or "dermatologist approved," really means a dermatologist puts the product on a patient's skin and nothing harmful happens such as irritation or break outs. With no standard test a product must pass to get this pledge of honor, a company can do any test it wants. There are times when a dermatologist will stamp their approval even if the product wasn't up to high standards. Sometimes it's not even a dermatologist. They just need to be a doctor, and a doctor that doesn't have the kind of knowledge about skin care that someone specific to the field would isn't very comforting. There is no law stating the products have to pass a test; they just have to be tested. Companies know these loopholes and fine print ways to get past certain information that you would find important when choosing a product.

So what are you left to believe when companies tell you something in regards to the validity and efficacy of their products? That is the answer—you can't believe everything you see in ads, whether that be on TV, the internet, social media, or billboards. Advertisers know the loopholes, and they know how to be sneaky to make the consumer hear what they want to hear to sell their product. Basically, any advertising out there is aimed at selling the product, not necessarily being honest or transparent. Too often, advertising companies know how to bend but not break the rules, and they take full advantage of that to sell, sell, sell. When it comes to looking for products or services for yourself, your best bet is to do some research. Learn about the ingredients in the products you are comparing. Do some digging because with the luxury of search engines at our fingertips, you can be knowledgeable about anything you want to make a purchase on if you just do some of your own research:

- **Fact-checking:** Read up on a product, read reviews from other consumers, and seek out your own research to find out if it's the right product for you and if it's worth the spending.
- **Product comparisons:** Explore and research all your options for your particular problem or the need you have to purchase this product. Compare pricing as well because it

could be on sale somewhere else or come with an offer.

- **Emotional awareness and mindfulness:** Pay attention to the emotions the advertiser wants you to feel and why. Try to keep a steady frame of mind, don't buy on impulse, and wait until after you go through your list to decide so you know it's something you have made a thoughtful decision on.

- **Decision-making skills:** Consider a pros and cons list, healthy discussion, or taking time to think before purchasing.

- **Boundaries:** It is a good idea to mute commercials or change the channel. Sometimes it is also healthy to take a break from the media hype. If you have a PVR that records your shows, you can skip through the commercials altogether.

Millions of people are on Facebook every day, and with the countless ads popping up on your Facebook feed that mislead you, someone is bound to get sucked into believing in some of them or wanting to believe something like a pair of underwear can suck in your fat and make you look like you've dropped 10 pounds overnight. There is a problem when you are just looking for the "easy way out." Advertisers have certain disclosure and truth to their advertising, but it's important to understand how they work with loopholes and fine print.

There are rules and regulations set out for advertisers to make sure the content you are seeing is somewhat valid. For example, in the United States, there is such a thing as the Federal Trade Commission (FTC) that governs any marketing or advertising. They help keep companies trustworthy by regulating how products are branded and what their labels claim. Such rules, regulations, and enforcement are very important, especially when it comes to child safety. The FTC helps keep certain industries from targeting children, like the tobacco and alcohol industry.

More and more ads seem to be targeting children and teens. They are easier to manipulate and tend to be more easily convinced. It is important to instill in our children the importance of having their minds made up, deciding things for themselves, and having a voice of opinion when they don't think something is accurate or they don't agree with something they see or hear. They are vulnerable to advertisements because they are more likely to accept them as reality without the critical-thinking skills necessary to ask important questions. Research shows the reward center in our brain is triggered when youth watch fast-food ads compared to other generic commercials. If they watch a commercial, they might not run out and go and get a greasy burger, but they're probably more likely to go thrashing through the cupboards, suddenly hankering for a snack. The primary focus is on consuming something unhealthy and processed. This unconscious effect these commercials have can be dangerous to weight gain and obesity.

Fast-food chains have managed to pull at the strong emotional associations that have been created through advertisements and other means. Children recognize brands and logos by the time they're two years old. It's very powerful, and once those emotional attachments are established, they're very difficult to get rid of (Garin Pirnia, 2019).

Fast-Food Chains

Fast food brings back childhood memories, memories of celebrations, or memories of great road trips. For many of us, fast food is associated with good times similar to other addictive substances. The advertisers of these big chain restaurants want to get to you emotionally. They want you to form an emotional attachment with their brand. Marketers try to get to your emotions by connecting their brand to basic human motivations—like accomplishment, belonging, and self-fulfillment—to encourage product sales. They also rely on humor and use it to make you laugh, and you will find that commercial more memorable than others because it gives you a giggle.

The resulting negative feelings that occur after you order your favorite greasy meal are not the focus when the decision is made to purchase fast food. Advertisers know what they're doing when it comes to selling a company's products and services, and fast food has the demographic pegged. Advertisers are paid to know what sells, and they don't think about people's feelings or consequences when they put their ads out. Advertisers know that, based on sales and other factors, people can't get enough of greasy, salty, sweet foods. If you ever watch commercials for big chain restaurants, it is always filled with happy, smiling people who are enjoying life and the food they are eating. Of course, a commercial isn't going to place any large people who are looking in the mirror, ashamed of what they look like. The advertisers will do anything to draw you in and give their products the most appeal.

Make sure when you eat out, you know what is in the food you are eating. The majority of restaurants, especially fast-food chains, must have a calorie display so you know how much you are consuming along with salt, sugar, etc. That is why it is best to limit your consumption of take-out food, even at a nice restaurant. Everything portrayed on the TV or internet is to make you feel like you want to buy that product. Fast-food chains tried to draw in children to their restaurants because they knew what a large demographic they were. If your child wants to go to a certain place to eat, chances are you are going to order from the same place. There are lots of advertisers that use celebrities to get people interested in their products.

Fast-food chains are probably the worst companies out there for misperceiving or convincing people watching that the food they produce is not as bad as it truly is. They are the worst at making you believe that the people in the ads are happy without a care in the world; meanwhile, there are people at home suffering from their relationship with food. If there are individuals out there who are trying to avoid seeing ads that have food in them, they better not turn on their TVs at all! There are actually around 50,000 different fast-food chains spread across the United States alone, and you can be sure to see an ad for one of them every time there is a commercial break or a chance to sneak in an ad on YouTube.

Fast-food restaurants are also aimed at being very inexpensive. Value and affordability are probably the two most important elements of fast-food marketing. In this tight economy, consumers would rather save a few dollars getting something that might not be healthier. It's not cheap to be healthy these days, and that makes it hard not to want to hit a drive-thru and get a whole meal for five dollars. When the biggest fast-food chain came out with ads introducing the dollar menu, everyone ate it up, literally. Most chains offer coupons and even apps now with deals and loyalty programs to suck you in.

They are also aimed at being quick and convenient. People always seem to be on the go, can't spare a minute in their hectic lives it seems. It's not that you don't know that fast food is not good for you. At that moment, you don't think about all the reasons you shouldn't eat at that fast-food place. You're just listening to your stomach. Some of the top reasons people choose fast food over a healthier alternative are

1. **It's quick:** Especially with most fast-food establishments having a drive-thru, it makes it quicker and easier than ever to get your lunch before your break is done. The microwave lunch you brought doesn't stand a chance though. By getting a quick fast-food lunch, you

can have time to enjoy what is left of your break.

2. **You don't feel like cooking:** It is much easier to stop in, grab a hot pizza, and have it ready for your family instead of coming home after a hard day's work and having to spend another hour in the kitchen, not to mention the dishes that will pile up along with it.

3. **When you are running late:** If you are like most people in the morning, you have hit the snooze button on your alarm clock too many times and are making a mad dash around the house to make sure you get ready on time. Even if you have managed to make time for a shower, the last thing you want to do is take time to prepare your breakfast or even your lunch for the day. It's much easier to hit the

drive-thru on the morning commute and have a fresh cup of coffee in tow.

4. **They are open late:** Early morning breakfast sandwiches and late night burgers make it way too easy to fulfill your hankering for a quick and satisfying stop. Whether you are in a hurry for work in the morning or you have been out too late having a night out, most fast-food restaurants and greasy diners are open for your pleasure.

Fast-food ads do affect healthy eating. You know how bad it is for you, but you keep coming back. You regret it right after, and your tummy might feel it, but you still always come crawling back because your brain remembers the happy feeling you get in your pleasure centers, and your craving must be met.

Advertisement and Body Image

Body image refers to a person's subjective perception of their body, which might be different when you compare it to how your body actually looks. Feelings, thoughts, and behaviors related to body image can have a major impact on your mental health and how you treat yourself. If advertisements are getting through on a subconscious level, what does that do for your self-image? When individuals with low self-worth or low self-esteem view advertisements that associate increased thinness with increased self-worth or are socially happy and accepted by their friends at their favorite fast-food restaurant, they often want to buy the products advertised. They also believe the people in the commercials are truly happy, even though they are having a burger and french fries.

The ads that we see on TV from a young age seem to be quite different when you compare males to females. Sadly, women are taught at a young age that their physical appearance is important. A study was done in regards to Saturday morning cartoon commercials, and 50% of commercials were aimed at girls about physical attractiveness, while none of the commercials aimed at boys referred to appearance (Kinsey, 2011). The diet industry must be doing something right because they're not losing customers. In fact, it's a billion dollar industry. You can't help but compare yourself to the ideal bodies that have been created. Women want to be thinner, and men want to be muscular, at least that is what has been engraved in our thought process. Men are targeted with unrealistic ways to look. Why is such importance put on something so unrealistic and sometimes impossible to attain? Body image is an important part of self-esteem. It's a realistic perception, and you deserve to value yourself whether you are overweight or underweight.

Body positivity has been top of mind recently, and that is a good thing for anyone out there who struggles with their self-image. Male, female, and youth all struggle in different ways with their physical appearance. It's okay to feel neutral or even indifferent about your body. You don't have to like everything about your body, and most of us don't.

Body positivity is important to loving yourself and being happy with who you are, even when your body goes through changes or you gain a couple of pounds. It's being happy with the person you are regardless of what society thinks you should look like. Thankfully, more and more companies are gearing towards more body positivity. Organizations are fighting against the way the media portrays the ideal body, makes others feel insecure, and promotes bad self-image by challenging how society views the body and promoting the acceptance of all bodies. Thanks to more of these organizations, others have been taking note and following in their footsteps. There are almost 15,000,000 #bodypositive posts on Instagram, and the body positivity movement is being showcased more and more (How The Beauty Industry Is Navigating Body Positivity, 2021). Body positive campaigns can create a sense of representation, which allows a sense of identity.

The fact that body diversity is being recognized is an important positive step forward. Self-care should focus on doing things that make you feel good about the body you have now. Show you respect your body with healthy food and take care of yourself. Exercise because it makes you feel good, inside and out. There are many other ways you can learn to accept yourself more by taking care of yourself and feeling like you have control.

Chapter 7: Controlling Emotional Eating

Food is nourishment for your body, and you need it to function, but it is also at the core of our identity, deeply associated with family, hearth, home, and community. Your favorite treat is usually purchased, you may have it when you want to celebrate, and some even avoid certain foods for religious reasons. Food choices can reflect our identity.

Your brain can associate eating a specific food to a specific context—for instance, popcorn and a movie, ice cream or a Slurpee on a hot day. This may cause you to crave that particular food the next time the same context comes around. The grocery stores know you are not just there to provide the basic needs for your family because they purposely market products in a way to get you to buy them, even if you may not need them. How many times have you left the market with a cart full of food when you had a list of items to fit a basket? It has been said that the majority of the healthier foods are in the perimeter of the grocery store, so try to avoid the inside shelves as much as you can. That is where most of the processed food and unhealthy snacks are.

Now that you have realized the concerns you may have with your emotional eating, how can you try and control it and eventually stop? If you want to make a change, first you must figure out what you are doing that should change. If you are eating to suppress your mood, or you have certain feelings and emotions that are triggering you to want to eat for comfort, there are steps you can take to lessen these triggers and be more aware of what is causing you to eat emotionally. Practicing mindful eating is the best way to attempt to stop emotional eating.

There are many ways you can respond to your emotions whether they are happy, sad, nostalgic, or angry. Look for other ways to connect with people or engage in activities that make you happy and can keep your mind off of turning to food. Try to ask yourself questions before you eat. Are you feeling hungry, or are you just upset? Will the food you are going to eat be healthy? Will the food satisfy you? Listen to your body more than your mind because if you aren't sure if you are really hungry, maybe you just need a glass of water or should go for a quick walk around the block to clear your head instead of going for that junk food. If you can put off eating for a while, then you know you weren't physically hungry, and if you can put it off with some other activities, it will help you from consuming those unneeded extra calories. Life can be so hectic and fast-paced, so it's important to remember to try to take the time to enjoy your food. Mindful eating is not difficult to do, and there are lots of ways you can make sure you are eating mindfully.

Mindful Eating

Mindful eating is something that could help anyone who wants to be more aware of what they are putting in their mouth and the effect of eating has in regards to surroundings, other distractions, and being more present. That's just what mindfulness is: being present in the moment. It is important to take advantage of the benefits your food can bring to your health. Be mindful not only in eating but of what you purchase at the grocery store and how you prepare your meals. When you eat mindfully, you are also less likely to indulge as often in those high-calorie, processed, greasy foods.

The Buddhist way of practicing mindful eating is to focus on sensual awareness of the food. It encourages you to pay attention to your food at every bite without any judgment. Your emotions don't come into play when you are mindfully eating. You are more in control of your eating, and your food isn't controlling you. Taking time to enjoy your food is what the Buddhists believe. There are six ways to help you be more mindful and take some time to enjoy your food:

1. **Engage your senses:** Look at your dish, smell the food, and take in the aromas for a few moments. Enjoy the texture as you take your bites.
2. **Take your time:** Chew your food thoroughly at least 20 to 40 chews. Your food will be digested better, and when you take your time, your mind has the ability to know you are full instead of eating so quickly that your brain

doesn't have a chance to catch up to your stomach.

3. **Know your cues:** Try not to wait until the last minute where you are famished. You tend to eat faster and might overeat. Instead, when you gradually feel hunger coming on, be prepared to eat soon.

4. **Appreciate your food:** Take some time to be thankful for the food you are about to eat, and appreciate its nutrition and the energy it will provide you until your next meal.

5. **Put down your cutlery:** Between each bite, take the time to set down your knife and fork to ensure you are not eating too quickly. Take your time chewing and savor the flavors.

6. **Be aware of your feelings:** Ask yourself if you are enjoying the food you are eating. Is it satisfying, or is it boring? If you find your meal

to be bland, maybe consider using more herbs or spices or finding a different recipe.

Mindful eating includes all aspects of your eating habits, including

- **How do you eat?** Slowly with intention.
- **Why do you eat?** You are physically hungry.
- **What do you eat?** Nutritious and filling foods.
- **When do you eat?** Don't wait until you're starving.
- **Where do you eat?** At home, most often.
- **How much do you eat?** Portion control.
- **Who do you eat with?** Mindful friends are best.

Keep a food journal and count your calories if you have to. Write down everything, even what you drink. Take pictures because your brain responds better to visuals; visual evidence is the best type and can trigger you to remember some of the ingredients in that meal. Know what you are putting in your mouth and how healthy or unhealthy it is. Everything is best in moderation. Keep your journal with you all the time so you don't forget to document anything. If you wait until the end of the day, it's easy to forget things like the creamer you might have added to your coffee. Try taking it day-by-day and document important daily feelings before and after you eat especially.

If you have your eating patterns and habits well documented, along with what you are eating, you can go back and read about what happened that day and understand what caused you to emotionally eat and the connection you have to food and your emotions. Make sure you write what you were doing while you ate so you can look back and reflect. If you notice you are distracted a lot when you are eating, maybe you can change those habits by sitting at the table without the TV or cell phone to distract you.

Additionally, keep track of your mood when you eat daily so you can understand how your mood might have affected what you ate. Since you are keeping track of your emotions, make sure you keep track of them before you eat and after you eat. If there are any discrepancies, you can take notes and reflect on them. What's your energy level? Does your digestion feel normal? How focused do you feel? Once you start going through your journaling, you might realize how much more you thought you were eating and how many calories you may be consuming that isn't necessarily required. You can figure out where to cut back and how to take different approaches towards your decisions for eating.

Change Your Habits, Change Your Mind

Keep snacks that you find difficult to stay away from out of the house. Out of sight, out of mind! When you head to the grocery store, make sure you aren't hungry. You're much more likely to buy something impulsively or purchase something more unhealthy because you are starving. Try to avoid buying groceries online or through an app if you can. It is also easier to buy impulsively.

If you feel like a snack, it's not a good idea to eat straight from the bag because you won't be mindful of how much you have actually eaten, and before you know it, the whole bag could be finished. When you prepare dinner, try to take the time to present it nicely. You eat with your eyes first, and even if you are preparing something healthy, your eyes will see how appealing it looks and enjoy it more. Try and keep your portion control in check; a portion is about the size of your fist. Start with a small portion as you take your time and hesitate before you go for seconds. You may realize that before you know it, you are satisfied and full.

Banish distractions. It might be habitual for you to turn on the TV and sit down to eat your meal, but it is best practice to have no distractions while you eat, especially if you are sitting down as a family. Understandably, life is busy, and if you have a hectic work schedule, you might be lucky to even get a lunch break. Your lunch might be quickly consumed at your desk while finishing reading your budget report. If you can try to take at least the time to enjoy your food, it would be better for your mindful eating.

Leave out the food commercials that consume the advertising world by using your PVR recorder if you can. That way you can just fast forward through all the commercials. You could also just mute them when they come on and use that as an opportunity to chat with your spouse, roommate, or company. Another easy step to take is to avoid watching too many commercials for restaurants or fast-food places, especially when you're trying to change your eating habits." With so many streaming companies out there, you don't have to be sucked in by commercials anymore. We have the ability to make healthy decisions, but it's much more difficult when the cues around us encourage otherwise.

If you find you are watching too much TV, try to fill your time with more activities to get you moving. If there are sports you especially enjoy watching on the TV, why not try getting out and learning them yourself? This doesn't mean you want to devote the rest of your life to getting into the Olympics, but it might be fun to join a club or a small league that isn't overly competitive. You can stay active, meet new people, and have fun distractions. Learning any new hobby or skill is a great way to kill time and stay distracted. Too much TV not only keeps us confined to sitting on the couch, but it can fill our heads with more unwanted stigmas and misinformed stereotypes on food, eating, weight, and other issues that you might be obsessing about.

Set goals and work to achieve them. Having something to work towards helps you look forward to your achievements and gives you focus. When setting goals, try to follow the SMART goals template:

S—Specific: Make your goals specific so you know exactly what you are trying to attain. For example, you could set out the days you want to work out, or you could set out a specific time of day you are planning on having your snacks. You can keep yourself on track better with specific goals for yourself and reflect on them later.

M—Measurable: If you want to be more measurable, you can set specific goals of weight loss. Maybe you plan on losing ten pounds in six months. You can be measurable by writing out your daily meal plan to know what your food goals are. If you need distractions, a good measurable goal is to meditate for ten minutes daily.

A—Attainable: You want your goals to be somewhat realistic so you can achieve them. If you set your goals too high, you might be setting yourself up for failure, which might lead to giving up.

R—Relevant: Make sure the goals you are setting are what you truly want to achieve. Don't leave any room for vagueness. Your brain will head to self-sabotage if you don't clearly understand what you want to achieve for yourself. Connect your goals to your life and what matters to you the most. Eating healthy and working out is a relevant goal because you want to be fit and feel good. Being more aware of your fitness goals ties into your emotional eating.

T—Timely: Set a reasonable amount of time you wish to achieve your goals. You need a mark of time to make sure you stay on track. You could write down how long you want to take to lose some weight if you have that as a goal, or you could give yourself a year to come up with better ways to handle your emotions that don't involve food.

What can you do to make cooking easier and take less time? Preparing dinner at home will save you a significant amount compared to eating out all the time. You will also save a ton of money. When you eat out, you are paying for much more than just the food. You are paying for the experience. Depending on where you go, you could be paying staff and other restaurant costs.

Prepare a grocery list based on what you have decided to make as meals for the week. When your meals are laid out for you, the temptation to eat out won't be so high. You know what you're going to make, so you don't have to worry about coming up with something last minute when you might just end up ordering out. Make sure you have plenty of cooking staples in your pantry: spices, herbs, oil, staple dry goods like pasta and rice, and staple canned goods like beans and tomatoes. You can buy your veggies pre-cut to save time on prep. If your potatoes or veggies take too long to cook, nuke them in the microwave to 'zap' some time off the cooking. Steaming veggies in the microwave is a quick and equally tasty method as well.

Another tip is to make extra of something the night before and plan to make another meal out of it. For example, one night, you could have salmon, broccoli, and rice. Make a bit of extra rice, and the next day you can make chicken or pork fried rice. A huge time-saver and a great investment, especially during the colder winter months, is a slow cooker. You can set it and forget it. Plop your roast in there with some vegetables and beef broth with your favorite seasoning, hit the timer for the right hours, and your dinner is ready by the time you get home!

Find out your triggers and foods that might bump you off track. You might have habits you have been taught since you were young, but you can turn them around. The best thing you can do for yourself is keep temptations out of sight. Don't buy them or have them in the house until you think you are ready to enjoy them in moderation. Eventually, you can make peace with food by challenging yourself with those foods you think are ' bad.' All these tips can turn into habits before you know it.

As mentioned in the first chapter of this book, too much fat, salt, and sugar can be bad for your overall health. When you are cooking at home, you are able to control all of those things much better. There are some ways you can cut back on fats, sugars, and salts.

Here are some ways to cut back on fat:

1. Meat is an important star of the show, but cut back on the fat by trimming off the fat of your beef and pork. Cut off any skin on your chicken or turkey, and try to choose leaner cuts of meat.
2. Try to use methods of cooking without oil, like steaming, and try to use healthy oils like avocado or olive oil when cooking. Butter and margarine can have high saturated and trans fats.

3. Try to use reduced-fat milk or cream when cooking. Plain Greek yogurt is a great alternative to sour cream.

Sugar is something we need little of daily; only about six teaspoons, actually. Too much sugar can cause tooth decay and excess weight gain, which leads to worse health issues like obesity and other diseases.

Here are some ways to cut back on sugar:

1. Fruit purees can be added to your yogurt or plain oatmeal to give it a bit of sweetness.
2. Try to use spices and other flavorings in your cooking instead of sugar. Orange or lemon zest or vanilla extract are good substitutions.
3. Dried or chopped fruit is a good alternative to adding sugar to your desserts or snacks. Anywhere you can save even a teaspoon will make a difference in the long run.

Even though sodium helps regulate blood pressure, overdoing it can lead to worse health issues in the long run. You shouldn't consume more than 5 grams per day. Taste your food often when you are cooking so you know if you need to add more. Wait until near the end to add more salt if needed. Other tips to reduce salt are

1. Gradually reduce the amount of salt you use in your diet, and your body will adjust to it better than drastically stopping your intake.
2. Fresh or dried herbs and spices are a great alternative to salt.
3. There is sodium-reduced soy sauce, canned vegetables, and broths that you can buy at the store. Try looking for any product that has reduced sodium.
4. Buy canned vegetables or tuna in water, not brine.

Use cooking as a way to get out of the house. Take time to pick your produce at the grocery store, or head out to your local farmer's market and find some quality produce and ingredients for your next dish. Cooking is a great way to socialize more and get closer to your loved ones. Use cooking time as a way of quality time. Some may feel like cooking is more of a chore than anything, but it is actually therapeutic and helps with boosting your mood. You can make it more fun if you do it with your partner or friends. Even cooking with your kids is a great bonding tactic. It is known to bring feelings of happiness and joy when you cook for others and get to see them enjoy the food you have prepared. It is important to feel more positive feelings when you think of food. It is better not to think of food as the enemy. Food has many ways of bringing people and families together through memories, nostalgia, and culture among other reasons.

There are many psychological benefits to cooking with loved ones:

- **You feel happy and connected to others:** Cooking can create bonds, and you feel like you are rewarded at the end of it. As humans, feeling connected is another human need. When you feel like you have supported someone and provided love through cooking, that connection is made and is strong.
- **It boosts self-esteem and makes you feel good:** When you prepare something yourself and afterward get to see how the person partaking is enjoying it, that is a great sense of accomplishment.
- **Cooking is a form of nurturing:** When you cook a meal for someone, you are providing

fuel for them, and it's that primal giving nature that is achieved. You have given a loved one something they need to survive.

- **It builds confidence:** When you try a recipe for the first time, maybe you don't get it just right. But you try again next time, and it just gets better and better, and you can even add your own substitutions, add some creativity and flair. That is such a good boost for your ego.

- **It can be therapeutic:** When you are in the kitchen, and you are enjoying all the smells coming from your food, that can sometimes trigger a memory of something meaningful from your past. Whether it be a smell that reminds you of a family member or a bonding experience you enjoyed, this is very therapeutic.

Cooking is a form of self-care because when you cook for yourself, you are sending a message that you care about yourself and you are important. You prepare nutritious meals for yourself, and that shows that you are also mindful of what you are putting in your body. Cooking does require quite a bit of focus, especially if it is something more challenging or something you haven't cooked before. That is a great way to stay mindful also, which is always good for your mental health. If you want to perfect some of your cooking skills, why not join a cooking class? It is another way to get off the couch and socialize and have fun. Cooking doesn't have to be a step-by-step, follow the ingredients to a tee kind of experience. Be creative and make it fun by exploring other ingredients and putting your own spin on your recipes.

Self-Care

A huge factor that can contribute to mindful eating is taking care of yourself. There are lots of ways you can reward yourself without food. Self-care is the best way you can reset and separate yourself from your emotional eating. Try to find other ways to feed your feelings: Join a sports team, book club, or find other activities to keep you occupied. Take some time to yourself to just unwind from the day-to-day, including your technology and social media. The majority of people seem to be overusing their cell phones. It's important to set boundaries for ourselves about how to use today's gadgets and media to our benefit, not become a slave of it. Having some guilt-free time to yourself, slowing down, and saying no to commitments that will push you past your limits can help bring you back to the present moment. You might just find you could use the time to reflect and unwind from your hectic day.

Here are some ways to practice self-care and reward yourself without food:

- **Pampering:** Take yourself to the spa for a pedicure or a massage. Take time for yourself and leave all your troubles behind. Sometimes getting a little me time is the best thing we can do for our mental health.
- **Try something new:** Try a spin class you might have never tried before or a dance class. Bring along a friend and make a fun day of it. Open your mind to new and exciting activities to feel good about yourself. You'll figure out what you love to do and break down old beliefs of who you are and what you can accomplish.
- **Reward yourself:** If you have been diligent at going to the gym and reaching some of your

fitness goals, or staying on your healthy eating path, you deserve a reward.

- **Meditation:** Relieve stress and clear your head through meditation. Even if you don't have a lot of time in your day, you might try to devote even 10 minutes when you are laying in bed first thing in the morning or during your morning shower. Try repeating some positive affirmations to get your day started on the right foot.
- **Listen to music:** Sometimes a touching song that makes you feel happy or motivated is just what you need. Maybe you have a good pair of noise-canceling headphones to listen to some soothing jazz or nature sounds.
- **Spa at home:** Take care of yourself at home if you don't want to spend a pretty penny. There are lots of great face masks you can buy at your

nearest drug store along with some great scented bubble baths or oils. Light a few candles and steep a nice herbal tea. Sounds good enough to try tonight?

- **Get active:** You have it in your mind to start working on your health, so if going for a hike, walk, bike, or to the gym is your way to destress and reset your emotional clock, by all means, kill two birds with one stone. You will feel great and you might start to see some impressive results in your waistline.

- **Read a book:** Choose books that put you in a good mood or motivate you. It will be nice to have the time alone and slow down your fast-paced life for an hour or two.

- **Organize your home:** Some people dread having to clean their home, but going through your closet or drawers can help clear your mind. When you don't feel cluttered in your personal space, your mind can feel more clear, and you will feel satisfied and accomplished.

Emotional Health

Emotional health isn't always about feeling good or being happy all the time, and it's not about never having negative emotions. It's about being able to experience, process, and respond to all the emotions that come with being human. It is important to have proper emotional health, so when something comes our way, we can solve it ourselves through positive thinking and good decision making. You will encounter many changes and challenges throughout your life, and it is important to be able to meet them head on and try to overcome them in a healthy way. Just as important as physical health is your emotional health. It can help you with your emotional eating by learning how to have good emotional intelligence.

You can always improve your emotional health by having the right frame of mind when it comes to challenges in your daily life. Having an open mind, being able to identify your emotions, and knowing they have value are important. It is also important to treat your feelings with importance and feel like your life has meaning to you. Eventually, you will be able to monitor your emotions, regulate them better, and have better outcomes.

Food only has power over you if you let it! Don't skip out on meals thinking you can beat your desires that way or save on calories. Your body still needs to be fueled. Don't be afraid, if all else fails, to seek professional help. Some counselors and therapists specialize in emotional eating and eating disorders to better assist you in your journey and goals. Some things you might want to ask your therapist are:

- What steps should I take to improve my emotional health?
- What are some other outlets to vent my emotions without involving food?
- Would medication will help me to be able to cope better?
- Should I see a therapist or counselor regularly?
- How does my physical health affect my emotional health?
- What stress management techniques would work best for me?

Along with therapy, some nutritional coaches can put you on the right eating path and help you along with information about what you should be putting in your body and what you should be avoiding. You can talk to your doctor about a referral to a good nutritionist, or you could seek one out online.

A nutritionist can help you with some of the issues surrounding food such as:

- **Connecting with your physical hunger signals:** Instead of associating your hunger as a bad thing, learn to listen to it and eat when you are hungry, not feeling a certain emotion.
- **How food matters:** Learning to listen to your body's hunger signals is critical for overcoming emotional eating. Skipping meals and not getting enough nutritional food is going to work against you.
- **Understanding your triggers:** When you know what triggers your emotional eating, you can create healthy, non-food strategies to overcome them. Don't be afraid of them because they can help you in the end.

- **Feeling your feelings:** Allow yourself to have uncomfortable feelings. Pushing them away is not going to make them disappear. Own them and learn positive ways to connect with them and yourself.

Speaking to someone who is a professional in the field of nutrition and health is going to make it easier for you to start to make the proper decisions and health goals. Nutritionists who have studied what a healthy diet consists of and how it can be worked into your new lifestyle can be a favorable resource for the road ahead.

Conclusion

So what are you going to do about the monthly budget meeting? You may have forgotten from before that that has crept up again. You have decided to make some positive changes and switch up some of your habits along with setting some goals for yourself. You still have to face the temptations you have no control over. Have you come to any conclusions about your emotional eating? If it started as a way to cope with your feelings but has become more of a crutch than you would like, then it's time for a change. With your emotions in check and the self-control you have learned in this book, you will have the skills to avoid certain situations and triggers. It's alright to create positive feelings around food. You don't always have to feel like eating is a bad thing. It's time to enjoy your food. Turning your food against you isn't working for you.

Habits aren't easy to break, and new ones aren't going to happen overnight. They take time. You have created some habits with your emotional eating, but they can be broken. The biggest arsenal you can carry is your awareness. That is going to be your biggest ally fighting against emotional eating. You have to be aware of your hunger and when it is pulling you in because of your emotions. Also, be aware of what you are putting in your mouth and how it can affect you after.

Keep yourself on track by avoiding those triggers that cause you to emotionally eat. Take yourself out of the equation when it comes to being overly tempted. There will be many setbacks, and it's important to learn from them and keep going. Talk to your friends and family and let them know about your new journey and the help you might need from them to stay focused.

Knowing some other underlying issues that have to do with your body and hormones plays a big part in understanding your body along with the emotional eating you might face. Hunger is driven by hormones in our body, and if any hormones are off track, it is best to know why and try to work with them to have an overall healthy lifestyle.

The decision you have made to change your habits is the first step in the right direction, and it might be a long road ahead. Don't overthink the future too much because you are going to need to focus and take it day by day. It is best to start gradually and start slow. Small changes can lead to bigger results. There might be a lot of work ahead for you when it comes to your habits and lifestyle.

What you think you know about emotionally eating might just be scratching the surface. It is important to keep a balanced life and remember your health is at the top of your mind, both physically and mentally. You know what is important in your life, and you need to stay connected to those things and surround yourself with positive people.

Constantly checking in with your emotions is important. When you think you might be hungry, make sure you are physically hungry. Be mindful and determine if you are hungry or upset, stressed, or bored. Don't be afraid to express yourself. Keeping your emptiness bottled inside will make it harder to cope with your emotional eating. You are not alone, and there is help out there as well as others that suffer the same obstacles with food. It might be hard to admit your struggle with food, but only you can choose to change it.

Afterword

Thankyou for reading "Stop Stuffing Your Face." I hope you enjoyed it. If you did and you have a moment, please leave a review.

Also please check out my previous book "How to Control Your Alcohol Consumption"

You can stay updated with my upcoming books on my social media pages and websites:

https://www.goodreads.com/author/show/1582808.Jason_Newman

https://twitter.com/Jason4Newman

References

6 ways to reward yourself without food. (2015 February 15). Paleo Leap. https://paleoleap.com/reward-yourself-without-food/#:~:text=%206%20Ways%20to%20Reward%20Yourself%20Without%20Food

11 simple health habits worth adopting into your life. (2020 November 2). Health Essentials from Cleveland Clinic.

https://health.clevelandclinic.org/11-simple-health-habits-worth-adopting-into-your-life/

A brief history of food preservation - The full dossier from DehydratorLab. (2018 July 16). Dehydrator Lab. https://dehydratorlab.com/history-of-food-preservation

Advertising laws and regulations. (2021). UpCounsel. https://www.upcounsel.com/advertising-laws-and-regulations

Andreas. (2020 August 1). *30 Major pros & cons of pesticides & herbicides.* E&C. https://environmental-conscience.com/herbicides-pesticides-pros-cons/#:~:text=%20Advantages%20of%20Pesticides%20and%20Herbicides%20%201

Axe, J. (2021 September 26). *The 30 most nutrient-dense foods on the planet.* Dr. Axe. https://draxe.com/nutrition/nutrient-dense-foods/

Bean-Mellinger, B. (2019 March 3). *The role of advertising in society.* Bizfluent. https://bizfluent.com/info-7736414-role-advertising-society.html

de Bellefonds, C. (2020 July 21). *15 Subtle signs you're eating too many processed foods*. Eat This Not That. https://www.eatthis.com/signs-eating-too-much-processed-foods/

Belsore, M. (2018 September 13). *10 Benefits of strength training besides building muscle*. Fitneass. https://www.fitneass.com/benefits-of-strength-training/#:~:text=Benefits%20Of%20Strength%20Training%201%20Increases%20Your%20Bone

Bidhuri, A. (2020 June 20). *Physical hunger VS emotional hunger: What is the difference?* PINKVILLA. https://www.pinkvilla.com/lifestyle/health-fitness/physical-hunger-vs-emotional-hunger-what-difference-543119

Brody, B. (2015 January 24). *The link between trauma and binge eating*. WebMD. https://www.webmd.com/mental-health/eating-disorders/binge-eating-disorder/features/ptsd-binge-eating#:~:text=Sometimes%2C%20a%20very%20bad%20%28traumatic%29%20past%20event%20causes

Byrne, C. (2021 October 21). *Why do we talk about emotional eating like it's bad?* Christine Byrne. https://christinejbyrne.com/emotional-eating-isnt-bad/

Capritto, A. (2019 September 27). *Why you should keep a food journal, and how to do it.* CNET. https://www.cnet.com/health/nutrition/stress-free-steps-to-keeping-a-food-journal/

Carnell, S. (2011 January 4). *Do you eat out of boredom?* Psychology Today. https://www.psychologytoday.com/us/blog/bad-appetite/201112/do-you-eat-out-boredom

Cathe. (2014 January 5). *Are there more overweight women or overweight men?* Cathe Friedrich. https://cathe.com/are-there-more-overweight-women-or-overweight-men/

Celes. (n.d.). *12 signs of emotional eating (And why it is bad for you).* Personal Excellence. https://personalexcellence.co/blog/signs-of-emotional-eating/#:~:text=12%20Signs%20of%20Emotional%20Eating.%201%20You%20eat

Cherry, K. (2020 November 21). *Why body positivity is important.* Verywell Mind.

https://www.verywellmind.com/what-is-body-positivity-4773402

Clark, J. (2009 June 15). *Can food make people happy?* HowStuffWorks. https://science.howstuffworks.com/life/food-happiness.htm

Crinklaw, W. (2019 December 6). *10 Reasons why people choose to eat fast food.* Society19. https://www.society19.com/reasons-why-people-choose-to-eat-fast-food/

Dryden-Edwards, R. (2017 August 18). *Emotional eating.* MedicineNet. https://www.medicinenet.com/emotional_eating/article.htm

Eknoyan, G. (2006). A history of obesity, or how what was good became ugly and then bad. *Advances in Chronic Kidney Disease, 13*(4), 421–427. https://doi.org/10.1053/j.ackd.2006.07.002

Emotional eating: What it is and tips to manage it. (2021 November 12). Cleveland Clinic. https://health.clevelandclinic.org/emotional-eating/

Emotional hunger vs. physical hunger. (2021 July 16). Modern Eve.

https://www.moderneve.org/blog/emotional-hunger-vs-physical-hunger

familydoctor.org editorial staff. (2020 June 20). *Mental Health: Keeping Your Emotional Health.* Family Doctor. https://familydoctor.org/mental-health-keeping-your-emotional-health/

Felman, A. (2020 July 9). *13 unexpected benefits of exercise.* Greatist. https://greatist.com/fitness/13-awesome-mental-health-benefits-exercise?c=765190705681#stress-relief

Ferguson, E. (2020 February 24). *10 Different ways to practice self-care.* Trendy Mami. https://www.trendymami.com/10-different-ways-to-practice-self-care/#:~:text=%2010%20Different%20Ways%20to%20Practice%20Self-Care%20

Fischer, E. (2017 October 4). *Eating and the cultural context of food.* The Great Courses Daily. https://www.thegreatcoursesdaily.com/itn-october-4/

Gibbons, A. (2014). *The evolution of diet.* National Geographic. https://www.nationalgeographic.com/foodfeatures/evolution-of-diet/

Gio. (2013 May 21). *What does dermatologist tested mean?* Beautiful with Brains. https://www.beautifulwithbrains.com/what-does-dermatologist-tested-means/

Girdwain, A. (2019 August 7). *Real talk: How much sugar should a healthy person eat in a day?* Well+Good. https://www.wellandgood.com/how-much-sugar-a-day/#:~:text=A%20good%20rule%20of%20thumb%3A%20Keep%20added%20sugars

Gunnars, K. (2018a December 4). *Leptin and leptin resistance: Everything you need to know.* Healthline. https://www.healthline.com/nutrition/leptin-101

Gunnars, K. (2018b December 4). *Leptin and leptin resistance: Everything you need to know.* Healthline. https://www.healthline.com/nutrition/leptin-101#reversing-resistance

Gunnars, K. (2020 November 5). *How much water should you drink per day?* Healthline. https://www.healthline.com/nutrition/how-much-water-should-you-drink-per-day#effects

Hanes, T. (2018 November 28). *Reason to live a healthy lifestyle.* Healthfully. https://healthfully.com/reasons-to-live-a-healthy-lifestyle-6749183.html

Harvard Health Publishing. (2020 September 7). *Are you getting essential nutrients from your diet? - Harvard Health.* Harvard Health. https://www.health.harvard.edu/healthbeat/are-you-getting-essential-nutrients-from-your-diet

Healthyplace.com Staff Writer. (2008 December 11). *Eating disorders: Body image and advertising.* Healthy Place. https://www.healthyplace.com/eating-disorders/articles/eating-disorders-body-image-and-advertising

Higgs, S., & Thomas, J. (2016). Social influences on eating. *Current Opinion in Behavioral Sciences, 9,* 1–6. https://doi.org/10.1016/j.cobeha.2015.10.005

Hormone Health Network. (2018 November). *Leptin | Endocrine society.* Hormone. https://www.hormone.org/your-health-and-hormones/glands-and-hormones-a-to-z/hormones/leptin

How did they cook food in the Stone Age? (2021). Philosophy-Question.com. https://philosophy-question.com/library/lecture/read/255808-how-did-they-cook-food-in-the-stone-age#:~:text=We%20know%20from%20historical%20research%20that%20the%20Inuit

How the beauty industry is navigating body positivity. (2021 July 26). The Dermatology Review. https://thedermreview.com/body-positivity-in-the-beauty-industry/

How to avoid eating free food from work. (2019 December 16). Cleveland Clinic. https://health.clevelandclinic.org/tempted-by-free-food-at-work-how-to-avoid-this-mindless-eating-trap/

Hughes, L. (2019 December 17). *How does too much sugar affect your body?* WebMD. https://www.webmd.com/diabetes/features/how-sugar-affects-your-body#:~:text=When%20you%20eat%20excess%20sugar%2C%20the%20extra%20insulin

Hunger: The 7 types & how to deal. (2017 September 10). The Leaf. https://leaf.nutrisystem.com/7-types-hunger/

Is obesity genetic? How obesity plays into your genes. (2020 July). Vitagene. https://vitagene.com/blog/is-obesity-genetic/

Kessler, A. (2019). *What these food cravings really mean.* Be Well by Alana Kessler. https://www.bewellbyak.com/writings/What-food-cravings-mean

Kinsey, A. (2011). *The negative influence of advertising.* Bizfluent. https://bizfluent.com/info-8196648-negative-influence-advertising.html

Kittelstad, K. (2019 March 30). *Examples of complex carbohydrates: List of common foods.* Your Dictionary. https://examples.yourdictionary.com/examples-of-complex-carbohydrates.html

Kwon, M. (2021). *Overnight oats.* Food Network. https://www.foodnetwork.com/recipes/overnight-oats-3416659#:~:text=Directions.%201%20Add%20the%20desired%20amounts%20of%20milk%2C

Lagerquist, R. (n.d.). *Is the human digestive system designed for meat?* Freedom You. https://www.freedomyou.com/is_the_human_dig

estive_system_designed_for_meat_freedomyou.aspx

Lehnardt, K. (2017 February 17). *96 Obesity facts, statistics, and more.* Fact Retriever. https://www.factretriever.com/obesity-facts

Levy, J. (2017 November 2). *Ghrelin: How to control this hunger hormone to lose fat.* Dr. Axe. https://draxe.com/health/ghrelin/

Lichterman, G. (2017 February 7). *Emotional eating and your hormones.* Hormonology. https://www.myhormonology.com/emotional-eating-and-your-hormones/

Liebig, R. (2013 February 26). *Water – Lubricates & cushions your joints.* Rhonda Liebig. https://rhondaliebig.com/water-lubricates-cushions-your-joints-more/#:~:text=Water%20makes%20up%20about%20two-thirds%20of%20our%20body

Lyngar, E. (2016 May 11). *The sexism of fat: It's easier to be a fat man than a fat woman.* Role Reboot. http://www.rolereboot.org/life/details/2016-05-sexism-fat-easier-fat-man-fat-woman/index.html

Marshall, M. (2016 January 25). *Is eating healthy really more expensive?* HuffPost.

https://www.huffpost.com/entry/is-eating-healthy-really-_b_9069318

Mayo Clinic. (2020 July 22). *Water is essential to your body*. Mayo Clinic Health System. https://www.mayoclinichealthsystem.org/hometown-health/speaking-of-health/water-essential-to-your-body

McAllister, J. (2011 June 3). *What do salt & sugar do to your body?* Livestrong. https://www.livestrong.com/article/461835-what-do-salt-sugar-do-to-your-body/

Migala, J. (2018 August 29). *The importance of healthy eating habits*. Everyday Health. https://www.everydayhealth.com/diet-nutrition/importance-healthy-eating-habits/

Miremadi, J. (2020 April 29). *Emotional eating 101 from a nutritionist who understands*. The Chalkboard. https://thechalkboardmag.com/wellness-toolkit-emotional-eating

National Institute of Diabetes and Digestive and Kidney Diseases. (2020 November). *Changing your habits for better health*. National Institute of Diabetes and Digestive and Kidney Diseases.

https://www.niddk.nih.gov/health-information/diet-nutrition/changing-habits-better-health

Nora. (2021 November 2). *FAQ: How many fast food chains are there in the United States?* The Infinite Kitchen. https://theinfinitekitchen.com/advices/faq-how-many-fast-food-chains-are-there-in-the-united-states/

Oglethorpe, A., Howey, N., & Edelstein, J. (2021 August 16). *The facts about emotional eating.* Real Simple. https://www.realsimple.com/health/mind-mood/emotional-health/emotional-eating#:~:text=Frequent%2C%20heavy%20emotional%20eating%20can%20be%20a%20serious

Peterson, T. J. (2015 October 13). *What is emotional health? And how to improve it?* Healthy Place. https://www.healthyplace.com/other-info/mental-illness-overview/what-is-emotional-health-and-how-to-improve-it

Petre, A. (2020a September 30). *What do food cravings mean? Facts and myths, explained.* Healthline.

https://www.healthline.com/nutrition/craving-meanings#:~:text=Your%20brain%20can%20associate%20eating%20a%20specific%20food

Petre, A. (2020b July 9). *What happens if you eat too much salt?* Healthline. https://www.healthline.com/nutrition/what-happens-if-you-eat-too-much-salt#long-term-effects

Persson, S. (2018 May 5). *Chemicals in food: Why they make you sick and how to avoid them.* Cancer Wisdom. https://www.cancerwisdom.net/chemicals-in-food/

Physical hunger vs. emotional hunger. (2014 February 21). Orchid Recovery Center. https://www.orchidrecoverycenter.com/blog/physical-hunger-vs-emotional-hunger/

Pirnia, G. (2019 March 18). *How fast food advertisements get under your skin, Whether you realize it or not.* HuffPost Canada. https://www.huffpost.com/entry/fast-food-marketing_l_5c890150e4b038892f493653

Preiato, D. (2020 May 4). *7 Ways that overeating affects your body.* Healthline.

https://www.healthline.com/nutrition/overeating-effects#1.-May-promote-excess-body-fat

Robertson, J. (2012 September 17). *Fast food and emotional eating.* Fitness Volt. https://fitnessvolt.com/4887/fast-food-and-emotional-eating/

Robinson, L., Segal, J., & Smith, M. (2019 June). *The mental health benefits of exercise: The exercise prescription for depression, anxiety, and stress.* Help Guide. https://www.helpguide.org/articles/healthy-living/the-mental-health-benefits-of-exercise.htm

Roeder, A. (2015 March 18). *Advertising's toxic effect on eating and body image.* News. https://www.hsph.harvard.edu/news/features/advertisings-toxic-effect-on-eating-and-body-image/

Rose, D. (2016 April 18). *The most powerful thing you should know about comfort foods.* MyFitnessPal Blog. https://blog.myfitnesspal.com/powerful-thing-know-comfort-foods/

Rosenbloom, C. (2009 June 30). *Calories, protein, carbohydrates and fat: how much do I need?* Canadian Living.

https://www.canadianliving.com/health/nutrition/article/calories-protein-carbohydrates-and-fat-how-much-do-i-need

Scott, E. (2021 January 5). *What is cortisol?* Verywell Mind. https://www.verywellmind.com/cortisol-and-stress-how-to-stay-healthy-3145080

Shah, R. (2020 September 10). *Evolution of the human diet: 80 Million years of eating.* Shortform. https://www.shortform.com/blog/evolution-of-the-human-diet/

Shoemaker, S. (2019 August 12). *12 Simple ways to drink more water.* Healthline. https://www.healthline.com/nutrition/how-to-drink-more-water#TOC_TITLE_HDR_3

Shulman, D. (2021 January 23). *Endocrine-related organs and hormones: Peptide YY.* Hormone. https://www.hormone.org/your-health-and-hormones/glands-and-hormones-a-to-z/hormones/peptide-yy

Shulman, D. (2022 January 23) *Endocrine-related organs and hormones: Ghrelin.* Hormone. https://www.hormone.org/your-health-and-hormones/glands-and-hormones-a-to-z/hormones/ghrelin

Smith, M., et al. (2021 September). *Emotional eating and how to stop it.* Help Guide. https://www.helpguide.org/articles/diets/emotional-eating.htm

Spritzler, F. (2016 March 7). *9 proven ways to fix the hormones that control your weight.* Healthline. https://www.healthline.com/nutrition/9-fixes-for-weight-hormones#TOC_TITLE_HDR_4

Superfoods: Broccoli benefits, nutrition and you. (2015 July 21). Superfoods Geek. https://superfoodsgeek.com/superfoods-broccoli-benefits-nutrition-and-you/

Szewczyk, J. (2018 July 16). *12 Little things you can do to make cooking at home easier.* BuzzFeed. https://www.buzzfeed.com/jesseszewczyk/how-to-make-cooking-easier

Thomson, J. R. (2017 July 17). *The very real psychological benefits of cooking for other people.* HuffPost. https://www.huffpost.com/entry/benefits-of-cooking-for-others_n_5967858ae4b0a0c6f1e67a15

TMP Admin. (2021 March 7). *Understanding the 7 types of hunger / The Mindfulness Project blog.* London Mindful.

https://www.londonmindful.com/blog/understanding-the-seven-types-of-hunger/

The truth about insulin and weight loss. (2021 January 25). Scottsdale Weight Loss Center. https://www.scottsdaleweightloss.com/the-truth-about-insulin-and-weight-loss/

The WCRF team. (2021 June 16). *5 ways to reduce fat, sugar and salt when cooking.* World Cancer Research Fund. https://www.wcrf-uk.org/our-blog/5-ways-to-reduce-fat-sugar-and-salt-when-cooking/

What are the 7 types of hunger and how to deal with them? (n.d.). Health Onlineium. https://health.onlineium.com/wellness/what-are-the-7-types-of-hunger-and-how-to-deal-with-them

Williams, L. (2019 May 19). *6 steps to the Buddhist practice of mindful eating.* Balance. https://balance.media/buddhist-mindful-eating/

World Obesity Federation. (2016). *Prevalence of obesity.* World Obesity Federation. https://www.worldobesity.org/about/about-obesity/prevalence-of-obesity

Yang. R. (2021). *Hormones: What are they and why do they affect our emotions?* Nannocare Period

Blog. https://nannocare.com/blogs/news/hormones-what-are-they-and-why-do-they-affect-our-emotions-1

Your Weight Matters Campaign. (2016 March 15). *Understanding the science of food addiction.* Your Weight Matters. https://www.yourweightmatters.org/science-food-addiction/

Zaz, I. (2015 March 24). *8 Ways to preserve nutrients in fruits and vegetables.* Bold Sky. https://www.boldsky.com/health/nutrition/2015/are-fruits-and-vegetables-less-nutritious-today/articlecontent-pf78792-066869.html

Printed in Great Britain
by Amazon